BREAST FEEDING

Macmillan Tropical Community Health Manuals
General Editor: Dr J. Grant, London School of Hygiene and Tropical Medicine

This series has been set up specifically to meet the needs of trainee and practising medical personnel in the tropical and sub-tropical developing countries. Some of the books will appeal to others involved in Community work — e.g. school teachers, public health inspectors, environmental health officers, and even literate parents. Early on there will be heavy concentration on aspects of care offering best prospects for improved standards of preventative treatment and therefore health in the community. Inevitably there will be strong emphasis on infant, child and mother care, as infants and children account for up to half the total population in some tropical developing countries, and more than half of the presentations for treatment.

Most titles will be short practical books written for trainee and practising doctors, nurses, auxiliaries, medical officers and assistants and other grades of health-care personnel engaged in frontline health-care delivery, often in small rural centres and sub-centres.

Other titles by G. J. Ebrahim in the Macmillan Tropical Community Health Manuals Series

Child Care in the Tropics	cased	ISBN 0 333 24038 3
	paper	ISBN 0 333 25361 2
Handbook of Tropical Paediatrics	cased	ISBN 0 333 24039 1
	paper	ISBN 0 333 25364 7
Practical Mother and Child Health in Developing Countries	cased	ISBN 0 333 24111 8
	paper	ISBN 0 333 25363 9
Care of the Newborn in Developing Countries	cased	ISBN 0 333 24112 6
	paper	ISBN 0 333 25362 0

The paperback edition of *Breast Feeding: the Biological Option* is published at a specially low price as a result of a subsidy provided by the Catholic Fund for Overseas Development.

BREAST FEEDING
the Biological Option

G. J. EBRAHIM

Published with the support of the
Catholic Fund for Overseas Development

First published 1978 by
THE MACMILLAN PRESS LTD
London and Basingstoke
Associated companies in Delhi Dublin
Hong Kong Johannesburg Lagos Melbourne
New York Singapore and Tokyo

Printed in Hong Kong

British Library Cataloguing in Publication Data

Ebrahim, G. J.
    Breast feeding. — (Macmillan tropical community series).
    1. Breast feeding
    I. Title
    649'.3   RJ216

    ISBN 0—333—23802—8
    ISBN 0—333—23803—6 Pbk

Contents

List of Tables

pg 83 photocopy

Preface

In the rural areas of the developing world, in urban slums and shanty towns infants who do not have access to their mothers' milk fail to thrive and even survive. Such communities constitute more than 80 per cent of the populations of the average developing country. And yet breast feeding has declined sharply in most such countries. The causes of this decline are several. Socio-economic development, rapid urbanisation, working mothers, have all been mentioned as possible causes. Yet they cannot be major causes because breast feeding is now making a come-back in many of the industrialised countries of the West where all these factors are present. In fact the two most outstanding causes of the decline of breast feeding are the high-pressure promotion of infant foods and the absence of a firm stand in favour of breast feeding by the health professions.

Breast feeding is only fleetingly mentioned during the training of most health workers. Many of the more popular textbooks assign only a small space to this aspect of child nutrition and rearing, with the result that the subject carries little intellectual appeal for the student. In recent years, however, a considerable amount of scientific research has helped to increase our knowledge of the nutritional and immunological properties of breast milk, and the biological importance of the mother's milk in the nurture of her offspring is better appreciated. One of the objectives of the book is to present some of these advances in a concise form in the hope that the subject will be taught and discussed more fully in the training programmes of the health and related professions.

When problems with breast feeding arise, intervention will be more successful if there is adequate understanding of the physiology of lactation and suckling. The first two chapters deal with these aspects of breast feeding.

As maternity services develop, more and more mothers will have their babies in hospitals, health centres and maternity units. When birth takes place at home in the traditional way, the birth attendant also helps with the establishment of breast feeding in accordance with the cultural practices of the society. On the other hand, in the modern obstetric unit the physician, the nurse and the midwife may unwittingly interfere with the establishment of breast feeding on account of the traditional routines of the maternity ward. These are discussed in Chapter 3 and suggestions are made for the successful establishment of lactation in the lying-in ward, and its maintenance later.

A knowledge of the mechanisms of synthesis and secretion of the various constituents of breast milk is necessary to appreciate the importance of the mother's milk in the nutrition of the infant. Chapter 4 reviews some of the new information in this respect and contrasts it with the possible effects of feeding with commercial formulae. The book was never meant to enter the controversy of breast versus bottle. And yet it was felt that the artificial feeding of infants should be put in the correct historical context, leaving it to the reader (and the teacher) to make comparisons and draw conclusions in group discussions. Chapter 5 provides a short history of artificial feeding, and points out that whereas artificial feeding first became possible because of technological developments in the beginning of this century, it did not become widely established until after the Second World War. As such, it is no older than three decades compared to the millions of years of human evolution during which the milk evolved with the species.

The last chapter discusses some of the nutritional, social and economic consequences of artificial feeding in the Third World. The problems of each developing country are unique and in a book of this nature only generalisations are possible. It is the author's hope that Chapter 6 will lead to discussions on the special problems within each country.

Finally, a word of explanation about suggested reading at the end of each chapter. A large bibliography would certainly have given the book a more 'learned' appearance. For example, more than 200 references were studied for the review presented in Chapter 4. Instead, the author opted for a short list of books and review articles. In the medical libraries of many poor nations only a few journals are available so that a large list of references will have served little purpose. On the other hand, by identifying key texts and reviews the author hopes to bring them to the notice of the interested reader.

G. J. EBRAHIM

Acknowledgements

The author and publishers wish to thank the following, who have kindly given permission for the use of copyright material:

R. M. Applebaum: Figures 1.3, 2.1, 2.2, and 3.7, from *Pediatric Clinics of North America*, **17**, 1 (1970), by permission of W. B. Saunders Company, Philadelphia, Pa, U.S.A.

F. E. Hytton and I. Leitch: Figures 1.4 and 1.5, from *The Physiology of Human Pregnancy*, 2nd revised edition (1971), by permission of Blackwells Scientific Publications Ltd.

S. J. Plank and M. L. Milanesi: Figure 4.5, from 'Infant feeding and Infant Mortality in Chile', *Bulletin of the World Health Organization*, **48** (1973) 203—20, by permission of the editor of *Bull. W.H.O.*

Brian Wharton and Howard Berger: Figures 5.1, 5.2, and 5.3, from 'Bottle Feeding', *British Medical Journal*, **1** (1976) 1328, by permission of Brian Wharton.

The author has made every effort to trace the copyright-owners of passages and illustrative material used, but if he has inadvertently overlooked any he will be pleased to make the necessary arrangements at the first opportunity.

Acknowledgements

The author and publishers wish to thank the following who have kindly given permission for the use of copyright material.

Chapter 1

Breast Feeding and the Mother – the Physiology of Lactation

Mammals have two characteristics – the presence of vertebrae and the nourishing of the young with milk from special milk-producing organs (mammae) of the mother. There are about 3500 known species of mammals. Naturally there is a wide variation in form, size and habit. Typical mammalian features are exhibited by man, dog, cow, rabbit and mouse. Less typical mammals are the water-dwelling whale and seal, the bird-like bat, the plated armadillo and the egg-laying duck-billed platypus.

In the evolution of mammals lactation is an attribute even older than gestation and the development of the placenta. For example, the most primitive order of mammals, the monotremes (the duck-billed platypus and the echidna or spiny anteaters), lay eggs which are received in the forepaws of the mother and placed between her curved tail and abdomen, where they hatch. Soon after, milk begins to appear in the 'milk area' which the young ones lick for nourishment.

In different mammals the number of the mammary glands and their location vary widely. Mammals who produce a large litter, e.g. the sow and many rodents, have as many as eleven pairs of glands. In pouched mammals, on the other hand, inguinal mammae occur. The location of the glands in a particular species depends upon their development along specific loci in the embryonic mammary ridges, followed by the disappearance of the intervening portion of the ridges. The organisation of the secretory apparatus within the mammary gland varies from one mammal to another. In the monotremes mentioned above, the 'gland' consists of a pair of pits which receive one hundred or more separate mammary tubules. There are no nipples. Milk is conducted from the openings of the tubules along hairs from which it is licked off or sucked by the nursing young. In the pouch of the kangaroo there are two nipples, each one capable of secreting milk of different fat content, so that the very young one is nursed with milk of high energy content in order to support rapid growth. After a certain time the fully grown baby attaches itself to the other nipple which will nourish him with milk more appropriate for growth at an older age.

1

For lactation to succeed, the first essential is that soon after birth the young should be able to find and suckle the mammary gland, and, second, the mother should accept the young. In many mammals the sense of smell plays an important role in both these processes. For example, studies in rats showed that immediately before parturition there is considerable increase in licking of the nipple line and the anogenital region. This behaviour decreases sharply after parturition. Instead the mother now licks the pups and it is thought that this licking behaviour is related to the formation of the mother—pup bond. In one experiment newborn kittens were removed from their mother immediately after birth and were fed by tube. After various periods they were returned to the mother. It was noted that after the 19th day the kittens did not seek the teat. It is believed that there is a critical period after birth in which imprinting can occur in the case of both the mother and the young one. Studies in goats and sheep have shown that the ability of an individual ewe to distinguish her own young by their smell is acquired within 20 to 30 minutes after birth.

Different species of mammals secrete milks of different composition (Fig. 1.1), indicating thereby that the food of the young has evolved

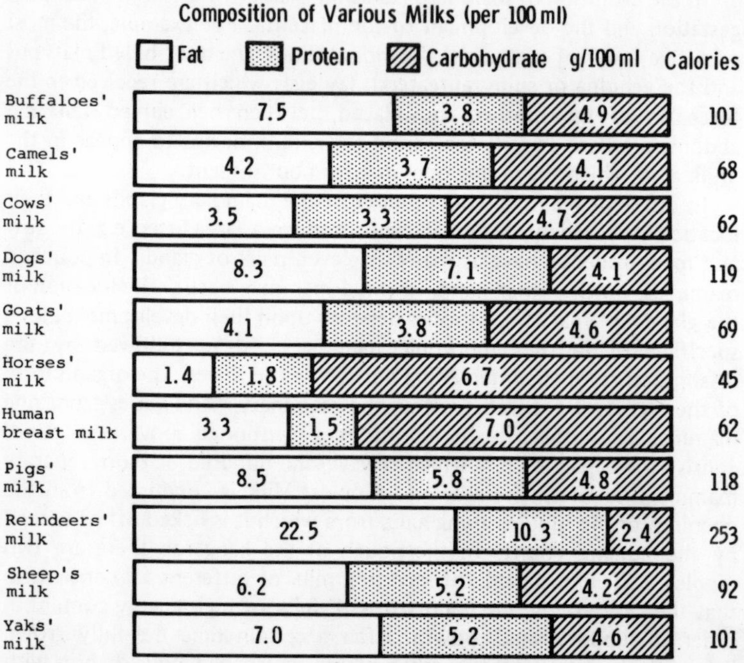

Composition of Various Milks (per 100 ml)

	Fat	Protein	Carbohydrate	g/100 ml	Calories

	Fat	Protein	Carbohydrate	Calories
Buffaloes' milk	7.5	3.8	4.9	101
Camels' milk	4.2	3.7	4.1	68
Cows' milk	3.5	3.3	4.7	62
Dogs' milk	8.3	7.1	4.1	119
Goats' milk	4.1	3.8	4.6	69
Horses' milk	1.4	1.8	6.7	45
Human breast milk	3.3	1.5	7.0	62
Pigs' milk	8.5	5.8	4.8	118
Reindeers' milk	22.5	10.3	2.4	253
Sheep's milk	6.2	5.2	4.2	92
Yaks' milk	7.0	5.2	4.6	101

FIG. 1.1 Composition of milk, various species

with each species. The energy and nutrient content of milk is related to the growth of the species. In general the energy content of milk secreted at maximal yield is about twice the calorific value of the body tissues of the mother oxidised during fasting. In most mammals this relationship does not change with species size. For the same species the milk yield is also related to the weight of the mother. The energy secreted in milk (kcal/day) varies with the body weight of the mother according to the equation Y (kcal/day) = 0.88 $W^{0.75}$ (Fig. 1.2). An interesting feature of all mammalian milks is concerning lactose, which

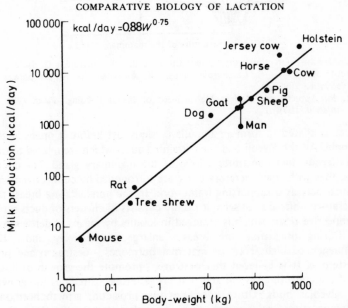

Milk yield (kcal/day at maximal yield) and body weight in mammals (From Payne and Wheeler's (1968) extension of Brody's (1945) graph)

FIG. 1.2   Relationship of body weight of the mother and calorie output in milk

is *the* milk sugar in all milks. Its concentration in the fat-free milk varies little from species to species, and over a weight range from mice to whales it is constant at 4—6 g anhydrous lactose/100 g milk. This may be due to the fact that in all milks lactose is osmotically a major component.

The Human Mammary Gland

The fully formed female breast is made up of 15 to 20 lactiferous ducts which branch repeatedly and drain secretory alveoli (Fig. 1.3). Each

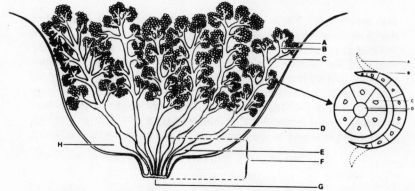

FIG. 1.3   Structure of the mammary gland

A. Alveolus. On the right, myoepithelial cell. B. Ductule. C. Duct. D. Lactiferous duct. E. Lactiferous sinus. F. Ampulla. G. Nipple pore. H. Alveolar margin.
(R. M. Applebaum, 'Modern Management of Breast Feeding', *Paed. Clin. of N. America* (1970).)

duct is dilated to form an ampulla or sinus just before it opens at the nipple. All the alveoli and their draining ducts which are related to one lactiferous duct constitute a lobe of the mammary gland. The ducts, together with their secretory units, are surrounded by connective tissue which acts as a supporting framework. In the non-lactating breast the secretory units are not seen; it mainly consists of clusters of ducts set in connective tissue which is arranged in lobules by means of dense septa.

During pregnancy the breasts enlarge progressively under the influence of high levels of maternal hormones — oestrogen and progesterone. It is believed that oestrogens promote the growth of ducts and the collecting system and that progesterone stimulates the growth of alveolar buds. Other hormones like prolactin, growth hormone, adrenocorticosteroids and the thyroid are also necessary for the optimal development of the secretory apparatus in the mammary gland.

There is a wide variation in the growth of the breasts during pregnancy. It is greater, as a rule, in younger women and in the first pregnancy. The lactational performance of the mother is also related to the growth of the breasts during pregnancy.

THE PHYSIOLOGY OF LACTATION

All women are not alike as regards their capacity for lactation. Some possess a much higher potential than others. In common with all physiologic functions the actual performance is not as great as the genetic potential, leaving room for 'physiologic reserve'. In the same woman second and later lactations tend to be more successful than the first, indicating that, as in all reproductive functions, 'trial runs' are necessary before optimal performance is achieved. In general younger women tend to perform better than older ones. To some extent this may be due to a kind of 'disuse atrophy' as measured by the time-lag between the mature development of the gland at puberty and its functioning after the birth of the baby.

From the physiological point of view lactational performance is related to nutrition, endocrine and psychological factors in the mother, as discussed below:

(i) *Nutrition*

During pregnancy maternal metabolism changes so that she lays down body stores of energy in the form of fat which is deposited in the subcutaneous tissue of the trunk and on the legs. In the well-nourished woman the increase in body fat amounts to about 4 kg, which is equivalent to a store of 35,000 kcal — enough to provide for lactation for four months at the rate of nearly 300 kcal a day. Thus the average woman enters the final weeks of pregnancy with a considerable store of food energy to act as a buffer against sudden deprivation of food (Fig. 1.4). Mothers who do not breast feed their babies will carry these extra stores of fat on their bodies unless they resort to dieting. In general, in the well-nourished community, mothers who breast feed are able to regain their figures more easily than those who do not. In the latter, as pregnancy follows pregnancy, there is a tendency to become obese.

As lactation proceeds the accumulated body fat is converted into energy in the milk. In a study of healthy women in Aberdeen it was

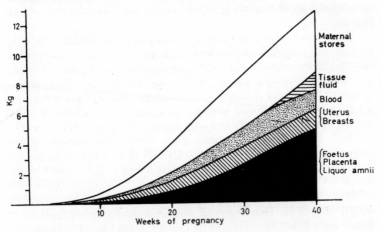

FIG. 1.4   The components of weight gain in normal pregnancy

found that during the period of lactation weight was lost at an average of 0.28 kg per week, even though the women were eating an average of 590 cal more than women in a control group who were not lactating. Assuming a milk output of 850 ml daily, which is what most healthy mothers are capable of, an equivalent energy loss of 600 cal has to be provided. Dietary energy is converted into milk with an efficiency of about 90 per cent. Based on these assumptions, and also on the fact that the body lays down stores during pregnancy, it is recommended that an additional 500 cal a day is an adequate supplement for a nursing mother.

The nutritional needs of lactation are chiefly for calories and not so much for proteins. Human milk is thought to have a protein content of 1.1 g/100 ml. This is calculated by estimating the nitrogen content of the milk, which is then multiplied by a factor of 6.25 to obtain the protein content. It is thought that this process overestimates the protein level by more than 20 per cent because of the contribution from non-protein nitrogen-containing constituents of the milk, and the true protein content of human milk could well be less than 1 g/100 ml. This small protein requirement of human milk can be easily supplied from a predominantly cereal-based diet so long as it provides adequate calories.

The high efficiency rate of conversion of food energy into breast milk in the mother, and the very low requirement of protein, added to the biological ability to store energy during pregnancy, enables mothers who are subsisting on marginal nutrition to breast feed their infants for prolonged periods. Mothers in prisoner-of-war camps have been reported to be able to breast feed their infants successfully. Similar descriptions about mothers in refugee camps also abound in the medical literature.

The concentration of various constituents of breast milk, like protein, fat, carbohydrate, calcium and iron, are little influenced by the nature and the amount of maternal diet within a wide range of intake and over a prolonged period of lactation (Table 1.1). Thus in New Guinea it was found that the composition of milk was much the same after 18 to 24 months of lactation as it was at 6 to 12 months. It is known that if the mother's diet is inadequate the output of milk will be reduced. Even then many studies have shown that mothers of low socio-economic class are able to secrete 400 to 800 ml of milk per day in the first year of lactation, the output falling to 200 to 450 ml per day in the second year.

When the diet during pregnancy is poor the mother will gain little weight (Fig. 1.5). Thus the *total* average weight gain in pregnancy in South India is 6.0 kg compared to 11.7 kg in the United Kingdom and 17.0 kg in the United States. In Tanzania the average weight gain in

TABLE 1.1   Composition of Breast Milk (g/100 ml)

	Protein	Fat	Lactose
Indonesia	1.67	3.3	7.14
New Guinea	1.01	2.36	7.34
India	1.06	3.34	7.47
Egypt	0.93	4.01	6.48
Pakistan	0.9	2.73	6.20
South Africa	1.35	3.90	7.1
England	1.07	4.2	7.4
United States	1.27	4.54	7.1
Australia	1.41	4.95	6.46

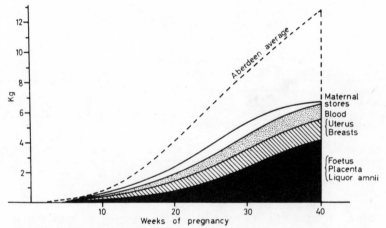

FIG. 1.5   Weight gain in pregnant Indian women in the low socio-economic class (Venkatachalam *et al.* 1960).)

pregnancy is 9.1 kg, and in Uganda it is 8.39 kg. Most of this weight consists of the weight of the baby and other products of conception, so that the true weight gained by the mother is very small. Such a mother will commence lactation with inadequate body stores of calories to fall back upon. In spite of this the milk output can be considerable. For example, in one study of South Indian women of low socio-economic group it was found that the average daily output of milk was 400 ml at the end of 18 months of lactation. Thus the child in his second year can be assured of almost one pint of milk daily in the poor circumstances of the rural household. It is likely that in such conditions the nutritional and energy cost of lactation is subsidised by maternal tissues. In one study 82 women of the lower socio-economic group in South India were followed from the 16th week of pregnancy up to one year after the birth of the baby. The average daily intake of food provided 1400 calories and less than 40 g of protein. The average weight gain in pregnancy was 6.5 kg, most of it (6.0 kg) comprising of the weight of the conceptus, so that immediately after the delivery the net increase in weight was found to be 0.68 kg. As lactation proceeded the women tended to lose weight for the first six months, after which the weight became stationary. The average weight loss in one year as compared to the initial weight of the mother was 1.5 kg, most of which (1.2 kg) occurred in the first six months after delivery. In spite of the loss of weight the secretion of milk was adequate to support the growth of the infants, who grew from an average weight of 2.90 kg at birth to 7.39 kg at the age of one year (Table 1.2).

TABLE 1.2　　Changes in body weights during pregnancy and lactation in women of lower socio-economic group in South India

	Initial wt	Wt before delivery	Wt immediately after delivery	Months after delivery			
				3 mths	6 mths	9 mths	12 mths
Number studied	82	82	82	72	59	60	56
Weight (kg)	41.91	48.53	42.59	41.27	40.55	40.41	40.36
Change from initial wt (kg)	—	+6.62	+0.68	−0.18	−1.33	−1.39	−1.61
Child's wt (kg)	—	—	2.90	5.02	6.60	7.05	7.39

(ii) *Endocrine factors*

The development, growth and secretory function of the mammary gland are dependent upon stimulation from appropriate hormones. In adolescent girls the breasts develop and grow to adult size under the influence of the sex hormones. In pregnancy there is further develop-ment of the secretory apparatus of the gland under the influence of high levels of circulating oestrogens and progesterone. Parturition triggers the secretion of prolactin from the anterior lobe of the pituitary, and under its influence the acinar cells of the mammary gland synthesise and secrete the various components of milk.

In all experimental animals hypophysectomy during lactation inhibits milk secretion. Lactation can be restored by supplying the necessary hormones, and in four species studied the following hor-mones were found to be necessary:

Species	*Hormones required*
Rat	prolactin and ACTH
Goat and sheep	prolactin, growth hormone, adrenal steroids and thyroxine
Rabbit	prolactin alone

In the human, endocrinologic control of lactation is by a complex combination of hormones. However, for all practical purposes prolactin can be considered the key lactogenic hormone in both initiating and maintaining milk secretion. Laboratory techniques of measuring prolactin have been developed comparatively recently. Since then, several studies have demonstrated the importance of prolactin in mammalian lactation. It has many similarities in structure and function to growth hormone and to the lactogenic hormone derived from the placenta. Together with other hormones like the adrenal steroids and thyroxine it forms the lactogenic hormone complex necessary for successful lactation.

In the non-lactating individual the secretion of prolactin is inhibited by a hypothalamic factor termed the 'prolactin-release inhibiting hormone'. This substance is synthesised in the hypothalamus and transported to the anterior pituitary in the portal system along the stalk of the pituitary. At delivery the inhibition of prolactin release is removed, resulting in the secretion of the hormone from the anterior pituitary. Recently it has been demonstrated that administration of the thyrotrophin-releasing hormone (TRH) results in elevation of blood levels of prolactin as well as thyrotrophin, suggesting that TRH could be a physiological prolactin-releasing hormone. It has also been shown that TRH improves milk output in women with declining lactation. Thus there are important possibilities for the clinical use of TRH.

Galactorrhoea is known to occur as a side effect of some drugs like reserpine and chlorpromazine. These pharmacological agents act on the hypothalamus, removing the inhibition exerted by the hypothalamus on the secretion of prolactin. These drugs have been used in the clinical situation to induce lactation in women.

The let-down reflex

Once the acinar cells of the breasts begin to secrete milk its continuing secretion and flow along the lactiferous ducts is maintained by a neuro-endocrinologic mechanism commonly known as the 'let-down reflex'. The nipple and areola are richly supplied with nerves. When the baby is put to the breast the tactile stimulation at the nipple during suckling results in afferent nerve impulses which travel to the hypothalamus. In turn the hypothalamus activates the anterior and the posterior lobes of the pituitary gland. Prolactin is secreted from the anterior lobe and under its effect the secretory activity of the acinar cells of the mammary gland is stimulated and maintained. At the same time oxytocin is secreted from the posterior lobe of the pituitary. It causes the contraction of the myoepithelial cells in the mammary gland, thereby propelling the milk along the duct. It is a common experience of many mothers that when the baby is put to the breast on one side, some milk may drip from the breast on the other side, and hence the term 'let-down' or milk-ejection reflex. Later, when lactation has been well established and the reflex mechanism has been reinforced several times over, many mothers experience a tingling sensation in the breast as feeding time approaches, or even on hearing the cry of the baby in the next room (Fig. 1.6).

The let-down reflex is the most crucial physiologic mechanism in successful lactation. Any factor interfering with the suckling at the breast by the infant will interfere with this mechanism and affect milk secretion, eventually causing the breasts to dry up. On the other hand, regular and repeated emptying of the breast by suckling will stimulate milk secretion and flow. In order to establish lactation the baby should be put to the breast as soon after delivery as possible, allowing time for the baby and the mother to recover from the rigours of labour. After this the breast should be offered 'on demand' in order to establish a flexible regime of feeding. Any 'top feeds' or feeds of glucose water will only serve to interfere with and weaken the let-down reflex by removing the stimulus of suckling, and should be avoided. The regular offering of the breast 'on demand' requires close mother–infant interaction which occurs best when the infant is nursed in the same bed in close contact with the mother, instead of in a distant nursery where easy access is not possible. When lactation fails, in most cases it is due to lack of adequate suckling stimulation through inadequate mother–infant interaction, or compliance of the mother with pressures to reduce the frequency or duration of suckling (e.g. the rigid routine of a maternity ward, or family pressures), or due to anxiety and uncertainty in the mother. The secretion of prolactin is proportional to the stimulation of the nipple and the areola. A confident approach in which the mother is encouraged to offer the breast readily without any reservation helps to overcome her anxiety and shyness, and also provides for proper development of the let-down reflex.

(iii) *Contraceptive effects*

In many peasant societies it has been noticed that, in the absence of any contraception, the interval between subsequent pregnancies is longer when a mother breast feeds her infant than when she does not. In the Philippines a birth interval of 24 to 35 months was found to occur in 51.2 per cent of the mothers who breast fed their children from 7 to 12 months. In Rwanda prolonged lactation gave rise to amenorrhoea in 50 per cent of the women for over 1 year and also contributed to a birth interval of 15 months as compared with a group of women whose babies died at birth and who therefore did not lactate.

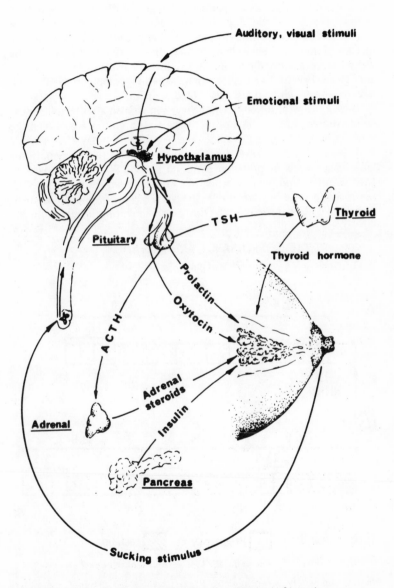

FIG. 1.6   The 'let-down' reflex and hormonal control of lactation

It has been estimated that the contraceptive effect of prolonged lactation, which is 'on demand' and unsupplemented, can amount to a reduction of as much as 20 per cent of expected births in areas of high fertility. In Chile the day of first ovulation after childbirth was investigated in 281 white women by using vaginal cytology, endometrial biopsy and basal temperature. It was found that when the women were nursing the infant on the breast exclusively, there was an average of 112 to 190 days to first ovulation, compared to 50 to 60 days in women who did not breast feed.

Measurement of blood hormone levels in women after childbirth has demonstrated that in the case of women who do not breast feed the levels of prolactin decrease rapidly and from the third day after delivery they are significantly lower than in the case of lactating women. In the latter, high levels of prolactin continue beyond 90 days post-partum. On the other hand, women who were breast feeding show low levels of oestrogen in spite of normal or high levels of gonadotrophic hormones. This would indicate that prolactin has an inhibiting influence on the

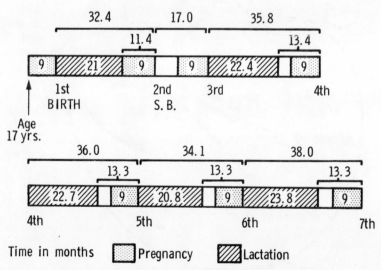

CYCLE OF PREGNANCY AND LACTATION
W. Africa

FIG. 1.7   Lactation, the central control of reproduction

In this community, where prolonged breast feeding was universal, the average birth interval was more than 31 months. But when a stillbirth occurred, the birth interval was reduced to 17 months in the absence of lactation.

synthesis of ovarian steroids. Since the secretion of prolactin is proportional to the duration and intensity of nipple stimulation, on-demand feeding and unsupplemented lactation is vital to cause delay in ovulation. These investigations demonstrate that lactation is not only an integral part of reproduction, in which parturition is but a milestone, but that it exercises a central control on reproduction (Fig. 1.7). Such a control is seen in many mammals and the best example is the kangaroo. When a mother kangaroo has a baby in the pouch, an ovum can get fertilised and will develop to the blastula stage, after which any further development of the fertilised ovum is arrested until such time as the baby has stopped suckling and has left the pouch. After this event the blastula will develop further, eventually producing an infant which is in no way different from that in which such an arrest in development did not occur.

PSYCHOLOGICAL ASPECTS

In many peasant communities prolonged breast feeding for periods up to 1½ to 2 years is the rule. If lactation lasts for such a long period it is more likely to do so because it is a process which gives satisfaction and pleasure to the mother and not because of the dictates of duty. The psychological responses of lactation, like nipple erection and uterine contraction, are similar to those of coitus. Some women are known to experience orgasm from breast feeding. The studies of Master and Johnson have pointed out that nursing women have a higher level of interest in sex than non-nursing post-partum women. Nursing women not only reported sexual stimulation from suckling but also were interested in rapid return to active intercourse with their husbands.

The mother's attitude is very much dependent upon the social and cultural milieu in which she has been brought up. If there is undue modesty and embarrassment at the thought of breast feeding, the 'let-down' reflex is likely to be inhibited. Similarly, in cultures which do not attach any stigma to breast feeding, the amount of suckling allowed is unrestricted and on demand, which is known to help milk production. Thus infants on an unrestricted feeding schedule are known to gain weight and grow faster than those on a rigid schedule. Similarly, those fed at short intervals grow better than those fed at longer intervals, demonstrating thereby that the frequency and duration of suckling are important in determining milk yield.

The mother's desire to feed her infant is aroused if there is a close physical contact with him. Infants who are nursed alongside the mother are fed more frequently than if they were kept in a separate nursery. The response of the baby is equally important. A lethargic baby sucks very little and thus does not stimulate milk production. In this respect

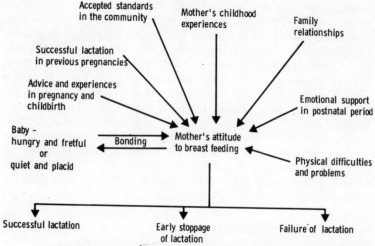

FIG. 1.8   Emotional and social factors influencing lactation

the amount of medication given to the mother is important. In the case of mothers who are heavily sedated with barbiturates during labour the infants may be drowsy for as long as 5 to 6 days after birth and are not capable of effective suckling.

The mother's own personality and life experiences are also important. Mothers with positive attitudes who react to their babies with joy and delight are on the whole more successful in breast feeding. Fig. 1.8 indicates the contributions of various psychological factors to the success or failure of lactation.

It is clear that a confident and cheerful approach from those who attend the mother in a friendly and sympathetic environment will go a long way in creating the emotional environment in which the physiological process of lactation can be initiated and developed.

Further Reading

1. Frank E. Hytten and Isabella Leitch, *The Physiology of Pregnancy* (Oxford: Blackwell, 1971).
2. 'Breast Feeding and the Mother', *Ciba Foundation Symposium 45* (N.S.), Elsevier; Excerpta Medica, North-Holland (1976).
3. S. K. Kon and A. T. Cowie (eds), *Milk: the Mammary Gland and its Secretion*, vols 1–2 (London and New York: Academic Press, 1964).
4. N. Newton and M. Newton, 'Psychological Aspects of Lactation', *New Eng. J. Med.* 277, 1179 (1967).

Chapter 2

Lactation and the Baby—the Physiology of Suckling

Suckling is the process by means of which the infant obtains milk from the mother's breast. It is not the same as sucking, even though some negative pressure is generated within the infant's mouth. During suckling the nipple is actually 'milked' between the infant's palate and the tongue by rhythmic movements of the tongue and the lower jaw.

In order to obtain his nutrition from the mother the baby should not only be able to find the nipple and suckle at it, but he should also be capable of swallowing the milk as well as digest and assimilate it. Physiologic maturity is necessary for the successful accomplishment of the different parts of the act. In the animal kingdom the initiative for suckling is always taken by the newborn. In the human, however, the mother must take the first step in bringing herself and her baby together.

Several reflexes enable the newborn to obtain milk from the breast. These are the rooting reflex, the suckling reflex and the swallowing reflex. The full-term baby, when lightly touched on the cheek near the corner of the mouth, will turn his head so as to bring his mouth to the object touching his cheek. This is the *rooting reflex*, which enables the baby to find the nipple when he is put to the breast. After the first few such experiences the baby begins to recognise the feeding situation, and will search for the nipple when he is picked up to be fed. In addition to the reflex mechanism itself other sensory stimuli such as warmth and smell must also play a part in enabling the infant to locate the source of milk. The sense of smell is important in the case of many lower animals. For example, if smell is blocked in baby rats (by instilling zinc sulphate in the nostrils) at the age of 2 days to 10 days they are unable to make successful contact with the teat and do not survive. Once the nipple is put into the mouth of such anosmic rats they can suck well and thrive, demonstrating that the only defect is their inability to find the teat. Recent studies in human infants indicate that the sense of smell may have a similar important role to play in enabling the infant to locate the nipple. When the breast pads of a mother are held near her infant the baby will turn his head towards them in preference to a clean pad held in a similar manner. This ability to distinguish the smell of milk can be demonstrated in a significant number of infants at the age of five days; by the 6th day many babies have a differential response between their own mother's breast pads and those of another. After the first few attempts at breast feeding the infant learns quickly and the mother will notice that she can generate a strong rooting reflex by stroking the infant's mouth with the nipple.

The *suckling reflex* is aroused when the baby first experiences the filling of his mouth, right up to the hard palate and the dorsum of the tongue, with the nipple or a nipple substitute. The full action in the reflex involves the jaws, tongue and cheeks (Fig. 2.1). The movements of the jaw enable the gums to press on the areola, squeezing the milk into the mouth. The tongue is at first thrust forward and then backward, compressing the nipple against the hard palate and creating a true 'milking' action. The muscles of the cheek create suction and

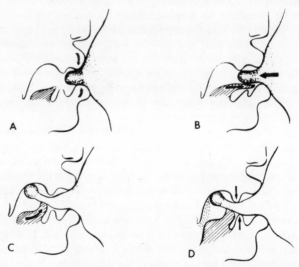

FIG. 2.1   The suckling response

A. The lips of the baby close around the nipple at the junction of the nipple and the areola.   B. The tongue protrudes to grasp the nipple.   C. The tongue pulls back bringing the nipple against the hard palate and the areola into the mouth.   D. Negative pressure is created by the action of the cheeks, the gums compress the areola and, with an active 'let-down' reflex, milk flows from the high-pressure system in the breast to the area of negative pressure in the baby's mouth.
(R. M. Applebaum, 'Modern Management of Breast Feeding', *Paed. Clin. of N. America* (1970).)

maintain a negative pressure in the mouth. Again, the infant learns from experience, and after a few days he becomes skilled at obtaining the milk from the nipple. The lips will now close firmly at the junction of the nipple and the areola, and the tongue will be thrust forward to grasp the nipple and bring it against the hard palate where the 'milking' can be done efficiently.

For a successful suckling reflex to be established the infant should be able to stretch the mother's nipple against the hard palate. A protractile nipple is vital for success in breast feeding, because only then is the infant able to take a proper grasp with his mouth and carry out the milking. In a large proportion of mothers who experience difficulty in establishing a good feeding response from their infants the nipples are not protractile, and on manual stimulation project forward by less than 2.5 cm, or not at all. In order to elicit a good suckling reflex, the *back* of the infant's mouth needs to be filled with the nipple, and hence the importance of adequate protractile nipples.

A rubber teat placed inside the infant's mouth can also evoke the suckling reflex similar to the one with the nipple. However, when the infant is fed with a bottle, the movements of the tongue and the cheek muscles are different (Fig. 2.2). There is a relaxation of cheek muscles, as opposed to contraction when suckling on the breast. The rubber nipple strikes the soft palate where the flow of milk causes the infant to gag. The tongue then moves forward and presses the teat against the

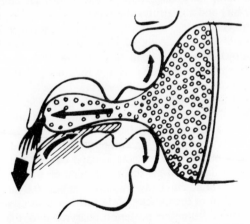

FIG. 2.2   Suckling response to feeding from a bottle

The lips open out to receive the nipple, and cheek muscles relax. The rubber nipple rests on the tongue, striking against the soft palate. The tongue moves forward to compress the rubber teat against the gums and the palate so as to control the flow of milk.

gums to control the flow of milk and to prevent flooding at the back of the mouth. Since the cheek muscles are in a relaxed position, the lips also are relaxed, making an O instead of compressing the teat as in the case of breast feeding. Thus less work is required to suck at the bottle. Introduction of the bottle at an early stage will create a learning response to it and weaken the baby's response to suckling at the breast. In some cases the desire to feed at the breast is also weakened. In the normal situation, however, the breast has the advantage over the rubber teat of the bottle in being able to elicit a strong suckling reflex except in the case of those mothers whose nipples are poorly shaped or retracted.

Between feeds milk secretion in the alveoli takes place at a constant rate. The passage of fat globules and protein granules from the cytoplasm of the alveolar cells into the duct lumen is passive by the process of dialysis. This form of secretion produces a watery milk of comparatively lower fat (2 per cent) and protein content. It travels down the ducts to the lactiferous sinuses and awaits ingestion by the infant at the next feeding. It is called the 'foremilk' and it constitutes about a third of the total milk volume available to the infant. When the infant suckles at the breast the secretion of oxytocin in the mother because of the let-down reflex causes the contraction of myoepithelial cells in her breast tissue. The alveolar cells are squeezed hard and the larger fat globules and protein particles are forced out into the duct system. The 'hind milk' so produced has a high fat content (4 per cent—7 per cent) and constitutes the remaining two-thirds of the milk volume. It mixes with the previously formed foremilk and increases its caloric content. Thus a strong suckling stimulus is necessary for a vigorous let-down reflex and milk flow. If the let-down is not strong enough the infant will consume only the foremilk which is insufficient to sustain him both in quantity and quality.

The composition of milk changes also during feeding. At the end of a feed breast milk contains 4—5 times as much lipid and 1.5 times as much protein as at the beginning. The concentration of lactose remains unchanged. These changes in the composition of milk during feeding occur regardless of the stage of lactation and control the satisfying of hunger on the one hand and the slaking of thirst on the other.

At each mouthful the baby swallows about 0.6 ml of milk. A co-ordinated action of the muscles of deglutition is necessary to convey the bolus of milk from the posterior pharynx into the oesophagus without aspiration into the respiratory passages. In the healthy full-term infant the *swallowing reflex* is well-developed, and suckling as well as swallowing present no problem. Oesophageal function, however, is not efficient in the first few days after birth, so that there may be an extremely rapid peristaltic rate, biphasic waves or even non-peristaltic

simultaneous contractions along the entire length of the oesophagus. As
the infant grows older oesophageal activity shows better co-ordination
during swallowing.

Recent studies indicate the presence of an upper airways reflex
mechanism which helps to prevent aspiration. In experimental animals
introduction of water or milk of other species in the upper airway
causes a period of apnoea and a swallowing action is evoked.
Introduction of normal saline or milk of the same species does not
produce such an apnoeic effect. Cow's-milk feeding in the newborn
activates this reflex. For example, it has been noticed that the infant
being fed cow's milk sucks continuously and breathes intermittently.
When the same infant is fed expressed breast milk from the same bottle
he sucks intermittently but breathes continuously. The breathing of the
infant is thus more regular when he is being fed breast milk, and such a
regularity of breathing cannot be demonstrated with cow's milk.

The neonate is a compulsive nose breather. Any obstruction in the
nasal air passages causes respiratory difficulty and restlessness. In the
case of the mother with retracted nipples the soft breast tissue will
press against the infant's nose during feeding, and cause obstruction to
breathing. Thus small retracted nipples are a common cause of
difficulty with breast feeding.

The reflex mechanisms mentioned above require a healthy and
vigorous infant with a well-functioning neuromotor system to bring
them into play. Sedatives and anaesthetics given to the mother before
or during labour can reach the infant, causing unresponsiveness to
environmental stimuli and inability to learn from the feeding situation
for several days. Moreover, if the vigour of his sucking is also
diminished, the let-down reflex will be weaker and the milk flow is
diminished. The barbiturates, the phenothiazines and the benzo-
diazepines all have such effects. It is not yet widely recognised that
local anaesthetics given to the mother are rapidly absorbed and cross
the placenta, so that peak levels are reached in the foetus within 9 to 10
minutes after a local anaesthetic block in the mother. Moreover, the
effects of such local anaesthetics persist for a long time in the baby,
causing serious problems with feeding.

Successful lactation depends so much upon the physiologic mechanisms of the mother working in synchrony with those of suckling in
the infant. It would not be correct to think of the process as merely a
mechanical one of secreting milk in the one and obtaining it in the
other partner. The mother and her infant work together as a 'diad'. One
is able to stimulate a response or mould it in the other. Thus not only
does the suckling stimulus by the baby result in the formation of milk
and in its ejection, but there is also evidence to show that the influence
of hormones circulating in the maternal blood stream moulds the nipple

to the suckling efforts of the baby. Moreover, the personalities of the mother and the infant come together in a mutually satisfying and pleasure-giving process.

THE NEONATAL GUT

In the full-term newborn the gastro-intestinal tract is well developed for the digestion and absorption of human milk. Several of the enzyme systems in the developing gut reach mature levels at or soon after term. Thus free acid can be detected in the stomach of the newborn within several hours after birth, and increases in amount in the first 24 hours. Pepsin secretion parallels the secretion of the acid and though less than the adult levels it is adequate for the pepsin digestion of milk. Tryptic activity is present in the pancreatic juice in a third of infants at 28 weeks' gestation. A tenfold increase in activity occurs between 28 and 36 weeks of gestation, after which the activity remains constant until term, followed by another tenfold increase between birth and the age of 9 months. Similarly, lipase activity is present at 34–36 weeks' gestation. It doubles by the time the infant is full-term and then a further tenfold increase in activity takes place between birth and the age of 9 months. In the mucosa of the small intestine α-glucosidases (maltase, sucrase, iso-maltase, amylase) are detectable in a three-month-old foetus, reaching maximal values by the sixth to eighth month of gestation. β-glucosidases (lactase) reach maximal value only at the end of normal gestation, though in the prematurely born infant develop-

TABLE 2.1   Development of digestive enzymes in the gut

	Foetus				Infant
	Before 28 weeks	28 weeks	28–36 weeks	36–40 weeks	Birth	Birth–9 months
Trypsin	–	First → detected in $\frac{1}{3}$ of foetuses	tenfold → increase	→	→	→ tenfold increase
Lipase	–		First → detected	Doubles →	tenfold increase
α-glucosidases	First detected at 12 weeks	→ maximal values →			
β-glucosidase	–	–	–	Maximal value	

ment of lactase activity occurs rapidly. Thus in the healthy full-term infant all the digestive enzymes are present in amounts adequate for the digestion of human milk (Table 2.1).

THE ASSIMILATION OF MILK

In the infant during the first few weeks of life there is hardly any urinary excretion of nitrogen, suggesting thereby that all the nitrogen consumed as protein in breast milk is in large measure utilised for building body tissues. Thus the infant does not burn protein for producing energy but utilises it solely for building body tissues. In this respect breast milk has a distinct advantage because of its unique amino acid composition. For example, several amino acids in cow's milk occur in amounts three to four times greater than in human milk. Also there is a difference in the proportions in which the individual amino acids are present (Table 2.2).

Many of the enzyme systems required for the degradation of various amino acids are not fully developed in the newborn so that infants, especially the premature, fed on cow's milk may show prolonged amino acid elevations in the blood lasting several weeks. Tyrosine, phenylalanine, branched chain amino acids and methionine are the amino acids which may be found raised in such situations. The clinical significance of such transient rises of amino acids is not fully known, but it is possible that intellectual deficits may arise, particularly in the case of the premature baby, on such feeding. Not only is the absolute amount of each individual amino acid important, but also the proportion in which various amino acids occur, as well as their relationship to the carbohydrate and other constituents of milk have a bearing on their utilisation. For example, the proportions of methion-

TABLE 2.2   Amino acid composition of human and cow's milk (g/l)

	Mature human milk		Cow's milk	
	Mean	*Range*	*Mean*	*Range*
Arginine	0.43	0.28—0.64	1.4	1.2—1.6
Histidine	0.24	0.12—0.30	1.2	1.1—1.3
Isoleucine	0.61	0.41—0.92	2.5	2.1—2.9
Leucine	0.97	0.65—1.47	3.6	3.2—3.9
Lysine	0.70	0.36—0.93	2.6	2.3—3.1
Methionine	0.12	0.07—0.16	0.8	0.6—0.9
Cystine	0.29	0.23—0.25	0.29	
Phenylalanine	0.40	0.24—0.58	1.8	1.5—2.2
Tyrosine	0.62	0.46—0.52	1.9	
Threonine	0.52	0.30—0.66	1.7	1.3—2.2
Tryprophan	0.19	0.14—0.26	0.6	0.4—0.8
Valine	0.73	0.45—1.14	2.6	2.4—2.8

ine and cystine in human milk are well adapted to the metabolic situation in the baby. On the other hand, cow's milk with its high methionine and low cystine contents tends to cause methionine accumulation when given in full strength and relative cystine deficiency when diluted. Because of these and several other aspects of the biochemistry of the newborn, breast milk remains the ideal food for the baby.

Further Reading

1. R. J. Grand, J. B. Watkins, and F. M. Torti, 'Progress in Gastroenterology: development of the human gastrointestinal tract — a review', *Gastroenterology*, **70**, 790 (1976).
2. N. C. R. Raiha, 'Perinatal Development of Some Enzymes of Amino Acid Metabolism in the Liver', in *Scientific Foundations of Paediatrics*, ed. J. A. Davis and J. Dobbing (London: Heinemann, 1974).

Chapter 3

Lactation and the Health Worker

There are three essentials for successful lactation, viz. (i) the parturient mother in whom physiologic mechanisms have caused the breasts to form milk, (ii) the infant with his in-born reflexes which enable him to obtain milk, and (iii) the immediate attendant of the mother, who can help to create the correct environment and act as a catalyst so that the physiologic processes in the mother and the baby can come together and operate in harmony. In most cases this is not difficult, as proven by the fact that a large number of infants are being successfully breast fed. After the initial few attempts both the mother and the infant learn to adjust to each other. The conditioning of their reflexes helps them to work in synchrony. The main contribution from the health worker is to provide confidence and emotional support to the mother, who is often torn by anxieties and fears of all kinds, and imagines difficulties.

The early days after the birth of the baby are crucial. As the milk is coming in, the mother is in a stage where she is recovering from one set of worries concerning the outcome of labour only to begin another concerning her ability to feed the baby and to be an adequate mother. Minor frustrations and failings take major forms in her mind. On the other hand, whereas most mothers are able to secrete milk, success in lactation requires attention to minor details like the way of holding the baby, the position of the mother during feeding, the protractility of the nipples, the baby's reactions and response to the feeding situation, and so on.

The first few attempts at feeding could be clumsy and may give rise to a great deal of maternal anxiety; but soon, with patience and perseverance, the responses of the baby and the mother get conditioned to each other. The mother will find that she is less clumsy at handling the baby. She will also notice that the baby has learned how to handle the nipple and to recognise the feeding situation. This process of learning and adjusting is quicker in a friendly environment with flexible routines, and where the mother has learned to trust the experience and competence of the health personnel caring for her.

23

The training of health workers in the management of lactation is most inadequate compared to the time spent on learning how to feed with a bottle. If the health attendant is to be able to manage lactation well, the primary requirement is for her to accept breast feeding as the normal scientific way of feeding infants. Her training should have convinced her that all other forms of feeding the infant are less than ideal and may even be hazardous. In addition to such a conviction, competent management of lactation calls for a thorough knowledge of the physiologic mechanisms involved, the effects of labour on the mother and the baby, the side effects of commonly used drugs such as ergot or analgesics and anaesthetics, and the emotional state of the mother after the birth of the baby. It also requires a knowledge of individual variations in the behaviour patterns of the baby and the mother, depending upon their personalities.

In recent years there has been an increasing emphasis on perinatal care, so that there is a trend towards institutional deliveries in almost all countries. Thus maternity wards and peripheral delivery units have the added responsibility of looking upon lactation as an integral part of the process of reproduction and promoting it in all possible ways. Routines and practices which help to reinforce the desire to breast feed, e.g. rooming-in, close body contact and flexible feeding routines, should be encouraged. Similarly, use of lactation sisters and voluntary helpers who can speak to mothers in the maternity ward and assist with minor problems should be supported.

There is more to breast feeding than what is written in the average textbook. Anthropological literature is full of examples of communities in whom, in case of the mother's death during childbirth, breast milk secretion is induced in the elderly grandmother or even young virgins by various means. The health profession tends to look upon such reports with scepticism, but now even in the Western medical literature there is a growing number of records of adoptive mothers who have been able to stimulate milk secretion in themselves by repeatedly and regularly suckling the infant at the breast. Considering what little is known about methods of inducing lactation or increasing the supply of milk in a mother it is surprising that such anecdotal reports have not been subjected to controlled clinical trials. In fact so little is taught and practised as regards stimulation of lactation and so well known are the established methods of 'drying up' the breasts after childbirth that it is quite obvious what the present trend in infant feeding is!

In theory every healthy woman who is able to conceive and carry a pregnancy to term should also be able to secrete milk. The only difficulties that can arise in this respect are the mother's own anxieties and fears, and faulty techniques of feeding. The fact that practically

every infant in the rural societies of the developing countries is fed on
his mother's milk points to the fact that these difficulties are not major.
With adequate training and experience the health worker should be able
to help the nursing mother to overcome the initial problems, if any, and
establish successful lactation. Minor problems like breast engorgement,
cracks and fissures in the nipples, the baby's apathy to suckle, etc., can
then be attended to with competence so as to build the mother's
confidence in herself and in those who provide medical care.

ANTEPARTUM PERIOD

Preparation of the mother for breast feeding should ideally commence
in the prenatal period when in individual talks and group discussions
she is helped to develop a positive attitude towards breast feeding. In
many cases it will be necessary to involve the husband or other heads of
the household as well, because very often the views and opinions held
by the mother are a reflection of those of the immediate family. When
the mother has a positive attitude and is favourably inclined towards
breast feeding the chances of success are better. The mother's attitude,
as expressed verbally shortly after delivery, is also related to success in
breast feeding. In one study 74 per cent of mothers with a positive
attitude had adequate milk by the fifth day as compared to 35 per cent
with doubtful and 26 per cent with negative attitudes. It is likely that
the mother who is not favourably inclined towards breast feeding will
not allow the infant adequate suckling at the breast. Also psychological
factors will interfere with the success of the 'let-down' reflex in her.
Unless breast feeding is common in a particular community many girls
will grow up without ever seeing a baby being breast-fed. Hence it will
be useful if some of the educational talks in the antenatal clinic are
given by mothers who have successfully breast-fed their own children,
and who can meaningfully discuss the details of the process with other
women. The experience of the mother in the antenatal clinic and during
childbirth is also important in developing a positive attitude. The
woman who maintains good health in pregnancy and has an uneventful
delivery, and with whom the health personnel are able to establish a
good relationship, is more likely to develop a positive attitude towards
breast feeding.

Some authors recommend physical preparation of the breasts for
lactation, and in the Western world several methods have been
advocated for the purpose. The Woolwich method, first suggested by
Waller, consists of teaching the mother to carry out manual expression
of the breasts during the last six weeks of pregnancy. The method is
based on the observation that the drainage of milk is more important
than its secretion by the acinar cells. The method aims at the expulsion

of early secretion, colostrum and cell debris from the duct system to facilitate adequate drainage. It is also claimed by the advocates of the method that by avoiding milk stasis and the accompanying inflammatory changes it prevents mastitis. In animal experiments it can be shown that raised intraductal pressure causes damage and involution of acinar cells leading to decreased secretion. However, many women find the massage of breasts offensive and would prefer to depend upon the infant to empty the breasts of these secretions by suckling. In such cases manual expression will be required if the breasts remain engorged in spite of regular suckling.

The other aspect of care of the breasts in pregnancy consists of preparation of the nipples. As we have seen, a protractile nipple capable of filling the back of the mouth is necessary for eliciting a proper feeding response in the infant. Tactile stimulation between the thumb and forefinger will cause the nipple to project in the majority of women, but in some it can retract. The Hoffman manoeuvre (Fig. 3.1),

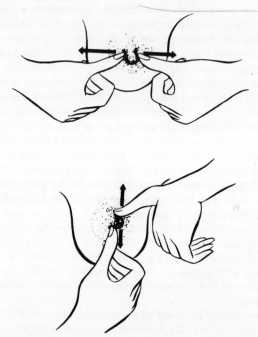

FIG. 3.1   The Hoffman manoeuvre for making the nipple more protractile

The nipple becomes erect with tactile stimulation from the thumb and the opposing forefinger, in the horizontal plane. The process is repeated in the vertical plane. The procedure, practised daily, helps to break adhesions at the nipple base, and makes it more suitable for grasping by the baby during nursing.

to be practised for several minutes daily, is recommended for such women in the last trimester of pregnancy. The movements are meant to break adhesions at the nipple base, so as to enable it to protract with tactile stimulation. The wearing of a nipple shield will also help to achieve the same purpose by exerting a continuous pressure on the tissues at the nipple base and making them more yielding. As pregnancy advances, physiological changes make the nipples more protractile, and some of the benefits credited to the above techniques may in fact be due to physiological factors. Thus in one study involving 170 primiparae, 34.7 per cent were judged to have defective nipples during pregnancy, but in the puerperium only 8 per cent were considered defective. In 104 multigravidae the incidence of defective nipples was 10 per cent during pregnancy and 4 per cent after the birth of the child.

The common anxiety most young women have is whether breast feeding will affect their figure by making the breasts more pendulous. There is no truth in this assumption. In the resting state the major proportion of breast parenchyma consists of the ducts which, together with fat and connective tissue, make up the total structure of the mammary gland. The increase in the size of the breasts during pregnancy is due to the growth and development of the acinar cells and the alveoli. When milk secretion begins the volume of milk present in the alveoli and the ducts adds further to the total bulk of the breasts. When the child is weaned and the secretion of milk ceases, the alveolar cells gradually disappear, being replaced by fat and connective tissue so that the breasts revert to their original size and shape, *provided that the connective tissue in the breast has not been overstretched.* The use of a well-fitting brassiere in pregnancy and during lactation prevents the breast tissue from being overstretched and maintains good shape. From another aspect of 'maintaining the figure' breast feeding holds a distinct advantage. It enables the mother to shed the weight gained during pregnancy and to return to her original weight easily and without strict dieting.

THE EARLY DAYS OF LACTATION

The early days set the course of lactation. If it gets off to a good start breast feeding is likely to remain trouble-free and mutually satisfying to both mother and infant. On the other hand, even small disturbances and difficulties at this stage can have major consequences.

The onset of milk secretion after the birth of the baby is a physiological event which seldom fails to occur. In contrast the establishment of successful lactation is a process which is dependent upon the constitutional, psychological and personality characteristics of the mother and the baby. Several post-partum events and routines of the maternity ward can either encourage smooth functioning or interfere with this process. Thus putting the baby to the breast soon after the delivery, and possibly even on the delivery table, is desirable, but a rigid ward routine may not allow it. Prelacteal feeds by the bottle are not necessary and, by causing the wrong kind of suckling response in the baby, are harmful, and yet are practised traditionally in many maternity units. Close and continuing contact between the mother and the infant creates the desire for breast feeding, but strict adherence to asepsis in the maternity unit may demand separation of the baby from the mother. Every baby has his own unique pattern of feeding, but rigid feeding schedules do not take such individual differences into account, so that there is interference with the smooth establishment of a feeding pattern.

The 'modern' maternity ward, especially in the Third World, has become a place where mothers come to learn about artificial feeding. Figs 3.2 to 3.6 are illustrations of some of the several ways in which mothers are initiated into artificial feeding through informal learning, observations and 'osmosis'. Such an experience gives rise to anxieties and doubts in their minds about the best way of feeding their infant. In such wards, when a mother wishes to breast feed, she finds that there are several 'difficulties' and it is only in rare instances that she can

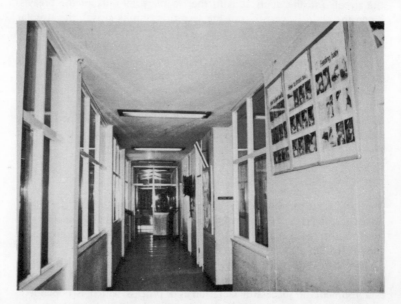

FIG. 3.2   Posters advertising artificial feeding in the corridor of the newborn nursery in a maternity hospital

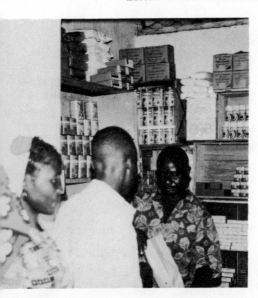

FIG. 3.3 The hospital store in a rural hospital selling several brands of artificial milk

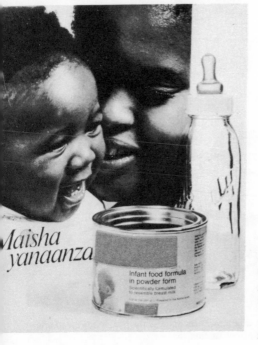

FIG. 3.4 The 'gift pack' given to the mother on the day after the delivery. The gift pack consists of a tin of powdered milk, a bottle and a glossy brochure.

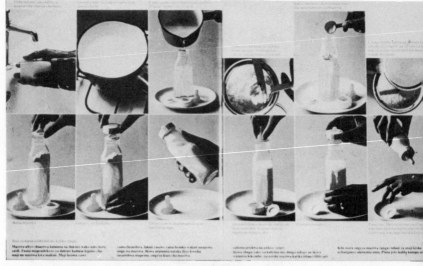

FIG. 3.5 Inside the glossy brochure there is a pictorial demonstration of preparation of the baby's feed

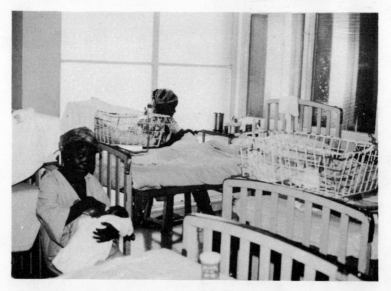

FIG. 3.6 The 'lying-in' ward where mothers practise the new lessons in artificial feeding

receive any real help with whatever minor problems she may have with nursing her infant.

SOME USEFUL HINTS

The earlier the suckling begins and the more complete the emptying of the breasts the more successful is the establishment of lactation. In the early days, therefore, the baby should be put to the breast for at least 10 minutes on either side, increasing the time to 20 minutes by the third day. Such a defined *minimum* period is important because the 'let-down' reflex operates 2 to 3 minutes later than the prolactin reflex. If the baby is removed from the breast too soon the reflex will be that much weaker. Just as suckling in the baby is affected by drugs so also the secretion of prolactin in the mother can be influenced by drugs like ergot given during the third stage of labour. In the same way the 'let-down' reflex can be inhibited by psychological stimuli like embarrassment at nursing, fear of discomfort, uterine contractions during breast feeding, or by actual pain from delivery. Careful attention to these details will enable a smooth suckling milk-flow act between the infant and the mother.

In the initial stages many mothers need to be shown how to hold the baby during a feed. As we have seen, for the baby it is not merely a question of calling up reflexes but that actual learning is involved. Such learning is facilitated by correct positioning. The baby should be held in the crook of the arm so that the head is free to move about and the back is supported. During feeding the baby turns his head slightly upwards as if he were looking up, and so the position should be such that the nipple is pointing at the baby's nose at the time of commencing a feed. During suckling, the baby should be held close enough for his chin to touch the breast. In such a posture the nipple is more likely to reach the top of his mouth, which is ideal for setting up the feeding behaviour. If the nipple is not well in the mouth, and the infant has to crane his neck forward, the nipple will come to lie on the tongue and the lower jaw instead. In this latter situation the baby can obtain very little milk from the nipple, which only teases and frustrates him.

For a large number of mothers once lactation is established and a pattern of feeding is set, there are no problems. In some, however, as milk secretion increases, certain difficulties arise. When secretion is in excess of what the infant can take, breast engorgement occurs. As milk accumulates in the duct system it causes back pressure so that circulation in the veins and the lymphatics becomes sluggish and there is oedema. The mother will then feel a sense of discomfort in the breasts. The best way of handling such a situation is to empty the breasts of milk by suggesting more frequent feeds, or by means of a breast pump or by manual expression. Within a few days, as the baby's milk intake increases, the rhythm between milk secretion and milk flow is established and the engorgement is relieved. Sore nipples, due to cracks and fissures, may be the first sign of breast engorgement. As the breasts become very full the natural concavity at the junction of the nipple and the areola is lost. When feeding, the infant finds a small nipple on which he cannot take a firm grip and has to struggle to keep it in the mouth. The 'chewing' action which ensues traumatises the nipple and causes cracks and fissures. Management consists of manually expressing a small amount of milk at the commencement of a feed. This will reduce the tension in the milk ducts and restore the concavity between the nipple and the areola. A very full breast may also press against the nose of the infant during feeding, causing 'air hunger', and the infant appears to 'fight at the breast' which is again a common cause of sore nipples. Infection may enter through fissures and cracks in the nipple and cause mastitis. All these conditions are preventable by a little care and alertness in the early days of lactation. If the baby is put to the breast more often and if the breasts are emptied by manual expression, drainage of milk is established and engorgement is fore-stalled. In summary, if the breasts are engorged the mother should not stop nursing, but on the contrary feed the baby more frequently. If at this stage the baby is not suckling well, breast massage and manual expression should be carried out to release the tension in the breasts.

In some instances the infant is not able to develop a proper feeding technique quickly enough. The mother complains that on being put to the breast the baby will commence feeding all right but will not go on. There are three possible causes of such apathy to feeding: (*a*) the nipple may not be well in the mouth, (*b*) the baby is satisfied soon, or (*c*) the milk may have stopped flowing, which is usually due to maternal anxiety interfering with the let-down reflex. Apathy can also occur when there is bad positioning during feeding or an insufficient hold on the nipple. Apart from apathy another cause of feeding problem in the infant is fighting at the breast. This is almost always due to difficulty in breathing due to an overfull breast impinging on the infant's nostrils, some form of nasal obstruction, or rarely due to the baby's upper lip riding up and blocking the nostrils during a feed (Fig. 3.7). The cause of apathy or breathing difficulty should be identified and corrected soon, because both can readily become habitual behaviour. Feeding by bottle as an interim measure is *not* the solution to these difficulties.

After the first week difficulties are rare. On discharge from the hospital the mother should be given a clear indication of how long breast feeding should continue. In many parts of the world infants are breast fed until they are 1½ to 2 years old, with of course suitable

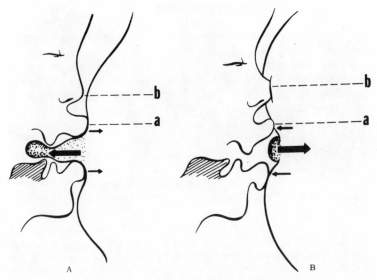

FIG. 3.7 Breathing difficulty during nursing

A. Normal. (*a*) The baby's lips can take a proper grasp of the nipple in the concavity between the areola and the nipple. (*b*) The nostrils are well away from the breast tissue so that breathing is free. B. Engorged breast or retracted nipple. (*a*) The baby's lips are unable to grasp the nipple, leading to repeated chewing movements and trauma causing cracked nipples. (*b*) The soft breast tissue presses against the baby's nostrils, causing difficulty with breathing.

solids being introduced from the age of six months onwards. When the baby is able to eat solid food well the mother may decide to take him off the breast gradually. On the other hand there is an essential minimum period of the first six months when breast milk should be the predominant food of the infant. Breast milk, as we shall see in Chapter 4, has properties other than purely nutritional, which protect the infant from infection and allergies. Such protection is necessary in the early months when the infant is vulnerable.

Once the process of lactation has been well-established its maintenance will depend upon the emotional and professional support the mother receives when she returns home with her newborn baby. Unfortunately, the tendency among health professionals in recent times is to be passive spectators and, at times, even active instigators of artificial feeding (Fig. 3.8). This is especially so in cases where the mother is in some kind of employment. It is easier and more fitting to the 'professional role' to write a prescription for the newest brand of powdered milk than to sit down with an anxious mother and painstakingly work out a schedule to suit her convenience. In

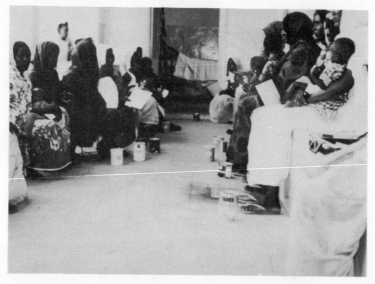

FIG. 3.8   Health workers as active instigators of bottle feeding

In this under-fives' clinic in the Sudan every mother attends with an empty tin to take home powdered milk provided free by an international agency.

communities where breast feeding is universal, and offered 'on demand', it has been observed that about a third of the total volume of milk ingested in the day, and a third of the total number of feeds in 24 hours are during the night between 8 p.m. and 6 a.m. Thus, even for a working mother, with adequate nursing breaks in the day, it should be possible to provide a considerable proportion of the daily requirements of milk for her baby with minimal supplementation.

A disastrous mistake is sometimes made when a nursing mother is admitted to hospital for an illness. The infant is not thought of by the admitting physician in a busy out-patient department, with the result that by the time the mother is discharged from hospital her milk has dried up and she is faced with finding an alternative as soon as possible. A similar situation can also arise when a sick infant is admitted to hospital without the mother. A little forethought in such circumstances can avoid a great deal of misery later.

To conclude, the health worker carries a heavy responsibility not only of ensuring the establishment of lactation at the time of delivery, but also of its maintenance through various family situations so that the infant can continue to derive the benefits of his mother's milk until such time as he is ready to be weaned on to solid food.

Further Reading

1. M. Gunther, *Infant Feeding* (Harmondsworth, Middlesex, England: Penguin Books, 1973).
2. M. Cameron and Y. Hofvander, *Manual on Feeding Infants and Young Children*, 2nd ed. (New York: United Nations, 1976).

Chapter 4

Breast Milk and Mechanisms of Secretion

The lactating mammary gland has a high metabolic activity, even greater than that of the liver, which is chemically the most active organ in the body. In full lactation there is a great uptake of substrate by the breast, which it utilises not only for the synthesis of the various constituents of milk but also for providing the energy required for such synthesis.

The acinar cells of the active gland show all the signs of intensive metabolic activity (Fig. 4.1). The nucleus is spherical and the cytoplasm has many mitochondria and ribosomes. Many of the ribosomes (up to 80 per cent of the total) are seen, on electron microscopy, to be bound to the rough endoplasmic reticulum (RER) where they carry out the synthesis of milk proteins. The Golgi apparatus, which is concerned with the storage, transport and excretion of the products of synthesis in the cell, is well-developed and can be easily identified. Some of the products of synthesis can also be seen. Thus there are protein granules and fat globules dispersed in the cytoplasm.

The various cell structures necessary for carrying out the synthetic activity develop within the acinar cells under the influence of the lactogenic hormones, and the process of synthesis itself is also triggered by sequential hormone action. The products of synthesis then pass into the duct lumen in two ways, viz. (i) an apocrine process in which large fat globules at the apical end of the cell are pinched off, sometimes together with portions of the cytoplasm, and (ii) an eccrine process in which passage occurs through the cell membrane without any 'pinching off' of portions of the cell.

MILK PROTEINS

The active mammary gland is very efficient at removing precursors of proteins and fats from the blood. Perfusion studies in the goat have shown that the mammary gland can remove 60 to 70 per cent of several amino acids and β-hydroxybutarate from the blood in one passage through the gland.

ULTRASTRUCTURE OF THE SECRETORY CELL

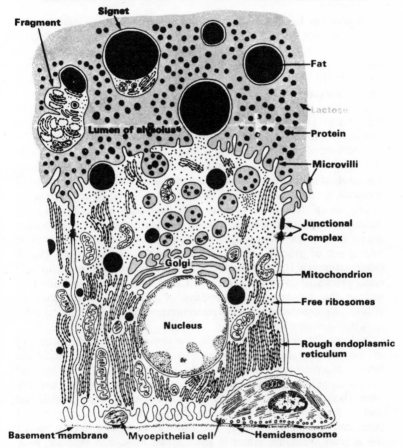

FIG. 4.1   Ultrastructure of the secretory cell

The milk proteins are formed in the ribosomes on the rough endoplasmic reticulum. The essential amino acids necessary for the process are derived from blood, whereas the non-essential amino acids are either derived from blood or synthesised in the mammary gland using carbon units from carbohydrate, fatty acid and amino acid sources. The protein molecules as they are formed aggregate into granules in the Golgi apparatus. Vesicles containing protein granules move to the apex of the cell and discharge their contents into the lumen.

There are three main classes of proteins in milk, viz. casein, α-lactalbumin and β-lactoglobulin. Human milk contains about 0.4 per cent casein. The remainder consists mainly of lactalbumin and lactoglobulin.

In addition to providing nourishment the proteins of milk are also associated with certain specific functions. For example, the several proteins of the casein group form miscelles with calcium and phosphate and are important carriers of these minerals, because the amount carried in this manner in milk greatly exceeds the quantities present in simple aqueous solutions.

It is now increasingly realised that the amino acid composition of the protein in breast milk is biologically the most suitable for the human infant. Several types of studies have been done to estimate the requirement of individual amino acids in infancy. In one type of study infants were fed mixtures of amino acids in various combinations, and the level of individual amino acids in the mixture which supported adequate growth was taken as the optimum level. In another study infants were fed a variety of milk formulae in quantities that maintained adequate growth and the concentration of the individual amino acids in the milks was then calculated. Using the data from these two types of studies, an Expert Committee of the World Health Organization (W.H.O.) made recommendations about the amino acid requirements of infants. In Table 4.1 data from these two studies, as well as the recommended quantities of individual amino acids by W.H.O., are compared with the concentration of the same amino acids in human and cow's milk protein.

Volume for volume, cow's milk provides not only larger quantities of the essential amino acids but also the proportion in which the individual amino acids occur is totally different (Fig. 4.2). Amino acid imbalance of such a nature affects the metabolism of protein, especially when there is coexisting immaturity of enzymes. It has been observed that in the average newborn infant the plasma amino acid levels fall immediately after birth. They rise again when feeding begins. Such a rise is brief when the infant is given breast milk. For example, peak levels of phenylalanine are reached on the 6th day and come back to normal on the 14th. When the infant is given cow's milk or any other high-protein feeds, the plasma amino acids remain elevated for several weeks or even months.

Each period in the life-cycle of an individual has its typical metabolic needs and physiologic characteristics. In the case of the neonate it is the inability to handle large amounts of protein, so that unlike the adult he cannot burn excess of protein to provide energy. With breast feeding there are, of course, no difficulties related to burning excess of protein or dealing with amino acid imbalance. And the reason for this is obvious. Human milk has a unique combination of amino acids necessary for this period of life, since the protein is

TABLE 4.1   Estimated requirements of essential amino acids and their concentrations in human and cow's milk protein

Amino acid	Amino acid mixture which will maintain adequate growth (mg/kg/day)	Amino acid content of various formulae which will maintain adequate growth (mg/kg/day)	The lower value (mg/kg/day)	Intake of 165 ml/kg/day		Suggested* pattern mg/g protein	Human milk mg/g protein	Cow's milk mg/g protein
				Breast milk (mg/kg/day)	Cow's milk (mg/kg/day)			
Histidine	34	28	28	36.3	156.75	14	20	27
Isoleucine	119	70	70	112.2	376.2	35	61	65
Leucine	229	161	161	165	577.5	80	90	100
Lysine	103	161	103	120.45	457	52	66	79
Methionine and Cystine	45 + Cys.	58	58	77	198	29	42	34
Phenylalanine and Tyrosine	90 + Tyr.	125	125	179.8	579	63	98	100
Threonine	87	116	87	82.5	270.6	44	45	46
Tryptophan	22	17	17	29.7	80.8	85	16	14
Valine	105	93	93	115.5	404.2	47	63	70

* Joint F.A.O./W.H.O. Expert Committee, 1973.

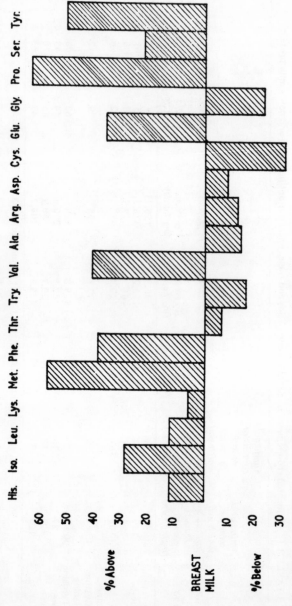

Comparison of the amino acid pattern of human and cows' milk protein using human milk protein as the standard. (The values, expressed as mg amino acid per g nitrogen in cows' milk, have been calculated as a percentage of those for breast milk expressed on the same basis.)

SOURCE: Food and Agriculture Organization of the United Nations, 1970.

FIG. 4.2   Comparison of the amino acid pattern of human and cow's milk

synthesised on the ribosomes in accordance with the genetically coded message for the species. The protein of breast milk is thus not only biochemically right, but also ideal from the biological point of view in that it is less antigenic. Moreover, because it is present in low concentration the gastro-intestinal tract of the infant is not flooded with large quantities of foreign protein substances.

LACTOSE SECRETION

The main substrate for the synthesis of lactose is uridine diphosphate galactose which is formed from glucose or galactose. The final step in the synthesis occurs in the lumen of the Golgi vesicles under the influence of the enzyme lactose synthetase which is present on the membrane of the Golgi vesicles. This enzyme has two components — an 'A' protein (galactosyl transferase) and a 'B' protein (α-lactalbumin) which is a major component of milk protein. The regulation of lactose synthesis is thus linked to the synthesis of milk protein and particularly to that of α-lactalbumin as shown in the diagram below:

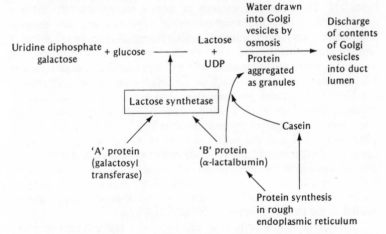

Both the components of lactose synthetase are under hormonal control. For example in explants of the mouse mammary gland it can be seen that administration of insulin, hydrocortisone and prolactin results in the synthesis of both the enzymes in the acinar cell.

The secretion of the major milk constituents is closely linked. Lactose synthesis is dependent on protein synthesis and, in turn, it determines the water and mineral contents of milk. The synthesis of lactose as we have seen takes place within the lumen of the Golgi apparatus and the vesicles carry it, together with aggregated protein granules, to the lumen of the alveolus where the contents of the vesicles are discharged. Hence for all practical purposes, lactose is formed 'extracellularly' and being unable to permeate cell membrane it draws water osmotically from inside the cell. It is the main mechanism by which the aqueous phase of milk is determined. As this phase of milk accounts for 95 per cent of milk it is also the mechanism by which the total milk yielded is determined.

Milk has the same osmotic pressure as plasma. Lactose and the main monovalent ions like Na^+, K^+ and Cl^- together are responsible for most of this osmotic pressure, and of these lactose accounts for about half. Thus the higher the level of lactose in milk the lower is the level of the various ions. Human milk differs from that of most mammals in that the concentration of lactose is high and that of the monovalent ions is low. The physiology of the baby is well adapted to its natural food, so that the human infant is a 'low-solute' organism and finds it difficult to handle large solute loads.

In the mammals the extremes of variations in the lactose content of fat-free milk are from 4 g per 100 ml in the dog and the elephant to about 7 g in man. In comparison the fat content can vary by almost thirtyfold. This relative constance of lactose secretion in the fat-free milk indicates that the mechanisms of synthesis and the enzyme processes are very much alike in various mammalian species. Lactose is also the predominant sugar in most milks with very few exceptions, like the monotremes and marsupials where the predominant sugars present are trisaccharides instead of lactose. Among the various sugars lactose is the ideal one because per molecule, and hence per unit of osmotic pressure, it provides nearly twice the calorific value than would glucose. The other advantages of lactose are that it influences the pH of the alimentary tract and the bacterial flora as well as the absorption of minerals. Furthermore, there is scientific evidence to indicate that lactose is essential for the synthesis of the galactolipids of the growing brain. For example, in several mammalian species the amount of galactose per unit weight of brain tissue in the offspring is closely related to the lactose content of the mother's milk.

Cow's milk is low in lactose and so in the manufacture of many infant feeding formulae, the first stage in the 'humanising' of cow's milk is to increase the sugar content. This is done either by adding more lactose or other sugars as shown in Table 4.2.

MILK FAT

Fat is present in milk as globules consisting largely of triglycerides surrounded by a hydrophilic surface layer composed of a mixture of phospholipids, cholesterol, vitamin A and carotenoids. Present evidence suggests that most of the long-chain fatty acids of the milk triglycerides

TABLE 4.2   The lactose content of human and cow's milks (expressed as g per 100 g of total solids) and the carbohydrate content (expressed as g per 100 g of powder) in some of the commonly used milk powders

	Lactose (g)	Sucrose (g)	Glucose (g)	Fructose (g)	Maltose Dextrins Starch (g)	Total (g/100 g total solids)
Human milk	56	–	–	–	–	56
Cow's milk	38	–	–	–	–	38
	(g)	(g)	(g)	(g)	(g)	(g/100 g powder)
Ostermilk 2	39	–	–	–	–	39
Cow & Gate 2	37	–	–	–	–	37
Ostermilk 1	64	–	–	–	–	64
Cow & Gate 1	63	–	–	–	–	63
S.M.A.	55	–	–	–	–	55
Nativa	54	–	–	–	–	54
Frisolac	57	–	–	–	–	57
Similac	54	–	–	–	–	54
Nan	64	–	–	–	–	64
Plasmolac	51	–	–	–	–	51
Humana 1	54	–	–	–	–	54
Humana 2	56	–	–	–	–	56
Almiron B	8	30	–	–	22	60
Milumil	23	28	–	–	13	64
Pelargon	29	14	–	–	17	60
Prodieton	23	33	–	–	20	66
Eledon	28	27	–	–	10	65
Pelargon	31	15	–	–	15	61
Pelargon	30	16	–	–	13	69
Guigolac	38	–	–	–	24	62
Farilacid	23	–	25	–	15	63
Milumel 1	32	15	6	3	5	61
Milumel 2	37	11	6	3	5	62
Lemiel 1	28	12	9	4	8	61
Lemiel 2	39	11	5	2	5	62

are derived from dietary fat and transported in blood to the breast as triglycerides in chylomicrons. Hydrolysis occurs under the influence of lipoprotein lipase present in the capillary walls in the mammary gland, releasing free fatty acids and partial glycerides which are taken up by the alveolar cells and re-esterified. In animal experiments it has been shown that prolactin administration can result in fatty acids from body stores being released for utilisation in milk secretion by the mammary gland.

The acinar cell can synthesise short and medium-chain fatty acids by a step-wise condensation of acetyl coenzyme A units up to a length of C_{16}. The esterification of fatty acids with glycerol takes place on the rough endoplasmic reticulum to produce fat droplets, which then coalesce to form globules within the cell cytoplasm. In the alveolar cell numerous fat globules can be seen scattered all over the cytoplasm. The smallest are present in the basal region of the cell and a progressive increase in size occurs the nearer the globules are to the apical membrane. The increase in size is due to the accumulation of freshly synthesised fat and finally the fat globule is released into the alveolar lumen by an apocrine process in which a portion of the cell membrane is 'pinched off' together with the fat globule.

Naturally occurring fatty acids contain 4 to 24 carbon atoms in a molecule. According to the number of carbon atoms present they are divided into long- (18 or more carbon atoms), medium- (8 to 12 carbon atoms), and short- (4 to 6 carbon atoms) chain fatty acids. The short-chain fatty acids are not abundant in food fats. The medium-chain acids are also not prevalent in food fats but are of interest because they are absorbed through the portal circulation instead of through the lymphatics by way of chyle formation. Long-chain fatty acids constitute the major proportion of fats in both human and cow's milk.

The fatty acids are also classified as saturated or unsaturated depending upon the presence of double bonds between the carbon atoms. The unsaturated ones may be mono- or poly-unsaturated depending upon the number of carbon atoms with double bonds. As a general rule the absorption of fatty acids in the gut is inversely related to the number of carbon atoms. The larger the chain the less efficient is the absorption. On the other hand, the more the number of the double bonds the better the absorption.

In all milks the triglycerides are made up mainly of long-chain fatty acids with 14 to 22 carbon atoms. Depending upon the species the fatty acids occur in varying quantities of saturated and unsaturated ones. In human milk they are 95 per cent long-chain and 5 per cent medium-chain as compared to cow's milk which has 83 per cent long-chain, 5 per cent medium-chain and the remaining 12 per cent as short-chain fatty acids.

The fatty acid composition of breast milk is dependent upon the source of fat in the mother's diet and the total amount of fat varies according to the adequacy of calories and other nutrients in her diet. Lipid content is also dependent upon the presence or otherwise of depot fat and its availability for the synthesis of milk fat. Mothers with inadequate nutrition tend to secrete milk with low-fat content in which short-chain fatty acids predominate. In one study it was found that when mothers were undernourished the quantity of milk fat fell to 1 per cent and even less, but the protein and lactose concentration was well-maintained. The principal fatty acids in these mothers had 10 to 14 carbon atoms in the chain compared to the well-nourished mothers in whom the fatty acids have 16 to 18 carbon atoms in the chain. The short-chain fatty acids (4 to 6 C) provide 5.3 kcal per gramme as compared to the medium-chain ones (8 to 12 C) which provide 8.3 kcal and long-chain ones (18 C or more) which give 9 kcal per gramme. Hence, even with the volume of milk secreted remaining constant, there can be a reduction of calorie content if there is qualitative change in the fatty acids of milk. A useful way of improving milk output and the quality of milk fat in the mother will be to improve her own nutrition, especially by supplementing with calories, a proportion of which can be in the form of edible oil.

The nature of body fat in the infant is largely determined by the quality of the fat in the diet. Tissue fat obtained by needle biopsy in infants shows a close similarity in the composition of fatty acids with dietary fat. Thus infants fed breast milk, cow's milk or a formula containing vegetable oils will lay down depot fat of different compositions (Fig. 4.3). This observation is important from two respects. The brain and the rest of the nervous system undergo rapid growth throughout early infancy. Fat is an important constituent of the nervous system and intake of biologically inappropriate kinds of fatty acids may have long-lasting effects on the growth of the nervous system. Second, as far as the intake of nutrients is concerned, the infant is dependent upon just one food source, viz. the milk. Unlike the adult who eats a varied diet and has several food sources providing a rich variety of nutrients the infant's choice is restricted to only those nutrients which are present in the milk with which he is being fed. There is virtually no margin of safety and any inadequacy in the milk will be translated into an altered composition of body tissues being formed at the time. Such a deficiency is then likely to be carried over to a future period when the required nutrients become available and the deficiency can be corrected. Whether such a restructuring of myelin can occur is not yet known, but present evidence suggests that it is unlikely to be so.

In order to avoid this difficulty the manufacturers of many brands of powdered milk modify the fat composition by removing butter fat from cow's milk and by substituting it with vegetable oils. In spite of such modifications serious differences between the fatty acid composition of human milk and powdered milks still remain. Table 4.3 compares the fatty acid composition of human and cow's milks with that of some of the more popular brands of powdered milks, as well as the commonly used vegetable oils in their manufacture.

Breast milk has an added advantage in that it is rich in lipase which is active even at low temperatures so that the digestion of milk fat begins long before the milk reaches the small intestine of the infant. In the young infant, free fatty acids are an important source of energy and the

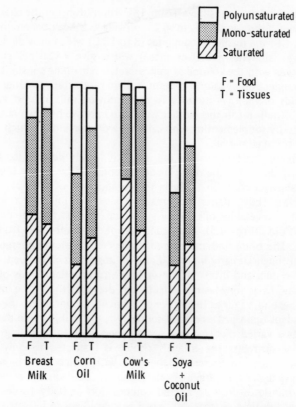

FIG. 4.3   Composition of depot fat and ingested fat in infants

Adipose tissue was obtained by biopsy in four groups of infants fed different formulae. Chemical analysis of the depot fat shows that the body fat tends to have the same chemical composition as that of dietary fat.

lipase of breast milk ensures that free fatty acids are readily generated from the infant's food. The effect of lipase is also dependent upon the chemical configuration of the fat being hydrolysed. For example, the most common of the saturated acids in both human and cow's milk is palmitic acid. In the case of human milk it is in the 2-position and is absorbed as 2-monoglyceride, whereas in cow's milk it is in the 1- or 3-position from where it is liberated as free palmitic acid in the lumen of the intestine, where it combines with calcium to form calcium palmitate soap and is excreted as such, resulting in loss of both fat and calcium.

The uniqueness of the fatty acids in breast milk, as indeed that of all the other nutrients, is ample evidence that 'adaptation' of cow's milk

TABLE 4.3   Fatty acid composition of human and cow's milks, commonly used vegetable fats in the manufacture of powdered milks, and several popular brands of infant feeding formulae

Fatty acid Nomenclature	Saturated							Unsaturated				
	4.0:8.0	Capric 10:0	Lauric 12:0	Myristic 14:0	Palmitic 16:0	Stearic 18:0	Arachidic 20:0	Palmitoleic 16:1	Oleic 18:1	Linoleic 18:2	Linolenic 18:3	Arachidonic 20:4
Human milk	0.46	1.5	7.0	8.5	21.0	7.0	1.0	2.5	36.0	7.0	1.0	0.5
Cow's milk	5.5	3.0	3.5	12.0	28.0	13.0	–	3.0	28.5	1.0	–	–
Oleo oils			0.2	3.3	26.0	20.0	trace		45.5	3.0	0.5	
Corn oil					13.0	4.0	trace		29.0	54.0		
Coconut	7.0	6.0	49.5	19.5	8.5	2.0	trace		6.0	1.5		
Soy				trace	11.0	4.0	trace		25.0	51.0	9.0	
Cotton				1.0	29.0	4.0		2.0	24.0	40.0		
S.M.A.		1.0	10	6	16.0	11	–	1	29.0	24.0	2.0	
Nativa		2.0	9.0	9.0	22.0	7.0	–	1	35.0	13.0	1.0	
Almiron B				<1	11	2	–	<1	27.0	58.0	2.0	
Farilacid		2.0	2.0	9	25	14	–	2	35.0	7.0	1.0	
Frisolac		<1	6.0	3.0	32.0	4.0	–	–	38.0	16.0	–	
Similac		2.0	19.0	7.0	9.0	3.0	–		19.0	40.0	<1	
Milumil		1.0	4.0	7.0	35.0	8.0	–	1	32.0	10.0	–	
Nan		2.0	4.0	11.0	31.0	9.0	–	2	24.0	16.0	1	
Humana 1 and 2		1.0	7.0	4.0	23.0	8.0	–	<1	44.0	13.0	<1	
Pelargon		2.0	2.0	8.0	24.0	11.0	–	1.0	30.0	16.0	1	

by dilution and addition of vegetable fats or sugars has no place in infant feeding and can give rise to unphysiologic combinations. For example, in one formula linoleic acid was added to defatted cow's milk in order to market a preparation with large quantities of polyunsaturated fat. Infants fed this formula developed a haemolytic anaemia. Investigations into the cause of the anaemia showed that the ingestion and absorption of large amounts of linoleic acid in the absence of vitamin E or other anti-oxidants led to the formation of peroxides which caused the haemolysis. There have been several similar instances of nutritional deficiency occurring in association with formulae which were 'humanised' in one way or another. One recent example is that of pyridoxine deficiency and megaloblastic anaemia caused by a formula which is now withdrawn. It is necessary to be constantly on the lookout for such dangers. The various nutrients in breast milk form a well-balanced mixture of fats, proteins, lactose, minerals and vitamins synthesised in accordance with genetic information coded in the alveolar cell and which has evolved with the human species. A low-protein content is possible because of the specific proportion in which the amino acids occur. Fatty acids occur in a ratio that will enable the baby to obtain adequate energy as well as to lay down myelin in the nervous system. The amounts of phosphate and calcium are in the correct proportion to promote adequate absorption. In spite of many advances in the sciences of nutrition and food technology commercial preparations remain only approximations of the natural product.

THE ELECTROLYTES IN MILK

In the cytoplasm of the alveolar cell the relative proportion of ions is similar to that inside all secretory cells. The 'sodium pump' on the basal membrane maintains the intracellular concentration of sodium (Na^+) relatively low and that of potassium (K^+) high, with a corresponding difference in the electrical potential on the two sides of the cell membrane. Both Na^+ and K^+ occur in the intracellular fluid as well as in the milk in the same proportion of 1 : 3, though the concentration of electrolytes in milk is lower than within the cell. Recent evidence suggests that the secretion of lactose is instrumental in determining the passage of ions into the milk and across the cell membrane. As we have seen, lactose is formed in the Golgi vesicles where its presence draws water into the vesicle by osmosis. The ions follow suit until equilibrium is established between the intracellular fluid and the contents of the vesicle. When lactose is discharged into the alveolar lumen from the vesicle water also gets drawn across and through the cell membrane. This biophysical process is largely responsible for the difference in the electrical potential on the two sides of the cell membrane. The variation in the lactose : ion ratio between species can thus be explained by differences in the rate of lactose synthesis, the permeability of the cell membrane and the electrical charge on the membrane.

Human milk is very low in electrolytes as compared to cow's milk. Table 4.4 gives the differences in the concentrations of the three main electrolytes of milk.

TABLE 4.4 Concentrations of main electrolytes
in human and cow's milks

	Human milk m.eq./l.	Cow's milk m.eq./l.
Sodium	6.5	25.2
Potassium	14.1	35.6
Chloride	12.1	29.0

Infants meeting their protein and calorie needs from breast milk obtain about 1 m.eq. of sodium per kg per day, compared to 4.8 m.eq. in the case of infants fed on full-cream cow's milk or unmodified dried milk powder. It is not widely appreciated that minerals are sometimes added to cow's milk during the manufacture of powdered milk in order to adjust the pH and make its composition stable. Sodium carbonate or bicarbonate is used in making some roller-dried and spray-dried milks, and sodium phosphate or citrate is added in the manufacture of evaporated milks. In some types of milks whey protein neutralised with sodium bicarbonate is used. When such preparations are fed to an infant the immature kidneys will be presented with a heavy solute load for excretion. In addition, the larger protein content of cow's milk also contributes to this excessive solute load. As a rough guide for calculating the renal solute load each gramme of dietary protein is taken as providing 4 milli osmols and each milli equivalent of sodium, potassium and chloride is taken as providing 1 milli osmol of such a load. The total available water for excretion by the kidneys (and carrying the solute load) is equal to the total amount ingested minus the insensible water loss and losses through faecal excretion. Fig. 4.4 gives the renal solute loads in the case of some of the common milk preparations in a 5-kg infant who consumes 200 ml/kg/day at varying levels of insensible water loss. It is clear that in the case of unmodified cow's milk and some of the commercial preparations the baby's renal concentrating capacity will be stretched, especially when the environmental temperature is high. For example, insensible water loss of 550 ml is not unusual in environmental temperatures of 90° F which are not infrequent in many tropical countries. If, in addition, there was any intercurrent illness as well, like fever or mild diarrhoea, such an infant

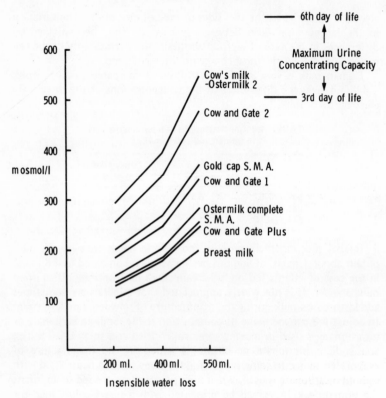

FIG. 4.4   Urine osmolar load in a 5-kg infant fed different formulae

will be at risk of hypernatraemic dehydration. Even in temperate countries several studies have shown that artificially fed infants have a higher plasma osmolality and sodium concentration compared to breast-fed infants (Table 4.5).

TABLE 4.5   Plasma osmolality, urea and sodium levels in breast-fed and artificially fed babies

	Breast-fed	Bottle-fed	Bottle-fed with additional solids
Number	7	14	26
Plasma osmolality (m.osm/kg)	283.7 ± 4.03	288.9 ± 7.30	288.9 ± 6.35
Plasma urea (mg/100 ml)	18.4 ± 7.81	53.0 ± 12.47	50.1 ± 10.87
Plasma sodium	135.9 ± 2.79	134.6 ± 1.87	135.2 ± 2.33

(Dale, G., *et al.*, 1975, 'Plasma Osmolality and Urea in Healthy Breast Fed and Bottle Fed Infants in Newcastle upon Tyne', *Arch. Dis. Childh.* **50**, 731.)

Any discussion on solute loads with powdered milk must take into account the effects of concentrated feeds. The type of scoop provided with the average tin of powdered milk lends itself to several difficulties in measuring the exact quantity of milk powder. In one study multiparous women, experienced health visitors and senior nurse midwives were asked to measure out the same number of scoops of powdered milk. When these quantities were weighed they were all unequal and many were far in excess of the manufacturers' figures! When measuring powdered milk with a scoop a slight change of manoeuvre, e.g. levelling with a knife as opposed to packing, can make a large difference to the quantity of powder measured.

When infants receive a heavy solute load in their feeds all the time and consequently develop a high plasma osmolality they are likely to feel thirsty more often and cry for a drink. If instead they receive another milk feed which is concentrated, a vicious circle gets established wherein concentrated feeds cause thirst and crying which leads to further feeding as shown below:

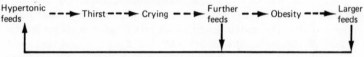

(Dunn, P., 1975, 'Subsidizing National Dried Milk', *Lancet* 1, 269.)

Many authors have warned of the dangers of such excess caloric intake in infancy, and in many instances obesity in the preschool period is noted to have its beginnings in the overfeeding of infancy.

THE MINERALS AND TRACE METALS

Calcium and phosphorus are the two major mineral constituents of milk. They are present in milk in concentrations exceeding those in blood plasma so that active transport mechanisms for their secretion must exist. However, virtually little is known about the secretory mechanisms except that those ions bind with casein to form micelles and that such binding occurs in the Golgi vesicles.

The absorption of calcium and phosphorus in the gut of the newborn is dependent not only on their concentrations in milk but also on other constituents, especially fats and vitamin D. Unabsorbed fatty acids tend to form soap with calcium, which is then excreted as such. Several studies on the relation of fat absorption to that of calcium have shown that there is a positive relationship between the excretion of fat and that of calcium. Even with high levels of calcium in the feed, inadequate absorption of fat can lead to faecal excretion of calcium soap.

Calcium absorption is also thought to be related to the proportion in which it is present with regard to phosphate. Human milk contains 33 mg of calcium and 15 mg of phosphorus per 100 ml as compared to cow's milk, which has 125 mg of calcium and 96 mg of phosphorus. Balance studies have shown that when infants are fed breast milk the retention of these minerals is in amounts equal to the estimated requirements for growth in spite of their comparatively low concentration in breast milk. This is partly because the two minerals occur in the correct proportion in breast milk and also because the fat in human milk is so well absorbed. Infants fed on unmodified cow's milk, either full strength or dilute, have low blood levels of calcium and in many of them the serum calcium will be low enough to cause tetany. In several commercial preparations the fat is now modified by replacing cow's milk fat with a mixture of vegetable and animal fats, and calcium as well as vitamin D are added so that tetany is rare, but in general, serum levels of calcium in breast-fed infants are higher than those of infants fed on most such formulae.

Breast milk was said to contain only small quantities of vitamin D and yet it is rare to see rickets in fully breast-fed infants even during winter months. The earlier assays of vitamin D were made on the lipid fraction of the milk, but recent work has demonstrated that unlike cow's milk most of the vitamin D in human milk is present in the aqueous phase as a sulphate. This water-soluble conjugate is present in concentrations of 0.91 to 1.78 μg/dl and is more than adequate for the infant's requirements of 10 μg per day.

The parts played by phosphorus and magnesium in neonatal physiology are not yet fully understood. In general, phosphate levels in serum tend to move in a direction opposite to that of calcium so that in tetany where calcium levels are low those of phosphate tend to be high. Some cases of tetany respond to the administration of magnesium and low levels of magnesium may have a causative role. With regard to electrolytes and minerals, establishment of homeostasis in the first few days of life is important, and colostrum is the main form of milk which helps to achieve it. The levels of the three minerals and the proportions in which they are present in human and cow's milk as well as some of the commercial preparations are given in Table 4.6.

Very little is known about the mechanisms of secretion of trace metals like copper, zinc and iron. In a study of fifty women between the 6th and 12th weeks of lactation it was found that the copper content of milk varied considerably among women and also within the same individual. The values ranged from 0.09 to 0.63 μg/ml. There is also a variation in the amount of copper secreted at different times of the day, the morning milk having a slightly higher copper content than the evening secretion. The secretion of zinc is more even, and does not

TABLE 4.6   The concentrations of calcium, phosphorus and magnesium in human and cow's milks and in some commercial preparations

Milk	Calcium	Phosphorus	mg/l Magnesium	Ca/P	Mg/P
Human colostrum	481	157	42	3.1	0.3
Human transitional	464	198	35	2.3	0.2
Human mature	344	141	35	2.4	0.2
Cow's milk	1370	910	130	1.5	0.1
Lactogen (1 to 9 dilution)	630	490	74	1.3	0.2
Ostermilk	560	460	49	1.2	0.1
Ostermilk 2	650	520	62	1.3	0.1
S.M.A.	560	440	53	1.3	0.1
Gold Cap − S.M.A.	440	330	53	1.3	0.2
Cow & Gate − Premium	550	400	45	1.4	0.1
Baby Milk Plus (1 to 8 dilution)	620	500	±	1.2	

show wide variations in the same individual. The mean value of zinc in breast milk is 1.59 ± 0.84 μg/ml. Breast milk also contains a ligand, a protein, which helps with the absorption of zinc in the infant. The iron content of milk is variable, the variations being present between women as well as in the same individual. The values range from less than 0.1 to 1.6 μg/ml. In the case of the healthy mother the average healthy infant receives 0.35 mg/kg/day of zinc and 0.05 mg/kg/day of both copper and iron.

ANTI-INFECTIVE PROPERTIES OF BREAST MILK

Mother's milk is not only a source of nourishment for the infant but also a strong antimicrobial agent because of the presence of several factors which act in synergism to form a biological system. For a long time epidemiological evidence has been pointing towards such benefits of breast feeding. At the turn of the century it was shown that the frequency of diarrhoeal deaths in British infants fed cow's milk was six times that of the ones fed on human milk. In 1951 a study of mortality and morbidity in 3266 British infants showed that both were lowest in breast-fed infants, highest in those who were bottle-fed and intermediate in those who were partly breast-fed. A similar study was carried out in Chile during 1969−70 when 1712 rural mothers were interviewed to assess the effects of feeding practices on the health of the infant. It was revealed that when bottle feeding commenced before the age of 3 months the mortality was three times that of breast-fed babies (Fig. 4.5).

In different mammalian species different physiologic mechanisms have evolved for the immunological protection of the offspring. In the

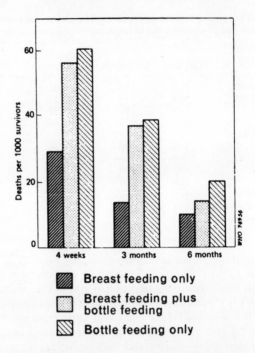

Breast feeding only

Breast feeding plus
bottle feeding

Bottle feeding only

Data from **PLANK, S. J. & MILANESI, M. L.**
Infant feeding and infant mortality in Chile.
Bulletin of the World Health Organization, **48** : 203–220 (1973).

FIG. 4.5   Mortality rate in the first year of life among infants surviving at 4
weeks, at 3 months and 6 months by type of feeding

case of the rabbit and guinea pig there is an outpouring of immune
substances, mainly gamma globulin, from the mother into the lumen of
the uterus during late pregnancy. Absorption occurs through the
membrane lining the yolk sac and transfer of immunoglobulin to the
foetus takes place. In the cow, goat, sheep, horse and pig there is no
such intrauterine transfer but instead the early secretion of the
mammary glands contain large quantities of antibodies which the
offspring swallows in the first few drinks. The gut is permeable in the
early stages, but after the first 36 hours resorption of immune
substances is no longer possible. The rat, mouse, cat and dog are in an
intermediate position. Transmission of antibodies from the mother to
the offspring takes place before as well as after birth. Resorption of
antibodies through the gut proceeds for a longer time, varying from 10

days in the dog to 20 days in the rat. In the human during pregnancy IgG passes from the mother to the foetus through the placenta. Antibodies against many common infections of childhood are carried in this component of immunoglobulins and provide passive immunity to the newborn in the first few months of life. Early studies on human colostrum did not show the presence of large amounts of IgG and it was thought that in the case of the human the only mechanism for transfer of immune substances was through the placenta. The importance of colostrum and breast milk as media for the carriage of immune protective factors went unrecognised until recently when more refined analytic techniques became available. It has been found that at birth colostrum contains 500 mg/100 ml of IgG; 48 hours after birth this value is around 100 mg/100 ml and 10 days after birth the mature milk has a value of 30 mg/100 ml. Studies at the National Institute of Nutrition in Hyderabad, India, have revealed that in breast-fed babies the serum levels of IgG are significantly higher at age 4–6 weeks compared to bottle-fed controls. Obviously the IgG in the colostrum and breast milk is responsible for this. It is possible that since the human infant receives a considerable amount of IgG transplacentally there is no urgency for large quantities to be provided through the breast milk immediately after birth, as in the case of the pig and calf. Instead it is received in small amounts over a period of time.

Breast milk also contains IgA, IgM and IgD. Of these IgA is in the largest amounts and has been shown to play an important biologic function. The concentration of IgA in breast milk is higher than that in the mother's serum, indicating active secretion rather than passive transfer. Moreover the configuration of the molecule in milk is different from that in serum. It is present as a dimer whereas in the serum it exists as a monomer. The two molecules of the dimer are joined together by a polypeptide chain, called the J chain. There is also a secretory piece attached to the molecule, which is a component of immunoglobulins found in secretions, and has the function of facilitating the passage of the molecule through the mucous lining. The composite molecule is more resistant than serum IgA to pH changes and enzymic attacks and is therefore active in the infant's gut. In several studies the antibodies carried in the IgA of the milk have been demonstrated in the stools of the breast-fed infant in amounts directly proportional to milk intake.

In the mammary gland the IgA dimers and the J chains are synthesised by the plasma cells found near the acini. The secretory piece is synthesised by the acinar cells and the entire molecule is put together during the passage through the epithelium on its way to enter the milk in the lumen of the acini. The concentration of IgA is high in the colostrum and decreases in the transitional and mature milk, but the total quantity secreted remains the same as the output of milk increases (Fig. 4.6).

Breast milk contains antibodies against many organisms, both viral and bacterial. In various studies antibodies have been demonstrated against tetanus, *Haemophilus pertussis, Diplococcus pneumoniae,* Shigella and *Escherichia coli* as well as against polio and coxsackie viruses. Most of these antibodies are of the IgA type. Since *E. coli* is an important pathogen in the neonatal period, and since a large proportion of IgA antibodies are against these organisms, a considerable amount of

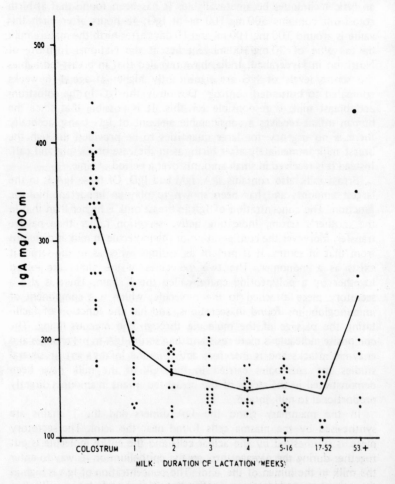

FIG. 4.6   IgA content of colostrum and milk

research has been done on the effects of breast milk on the colonisation of the neonatal gut by *E. coli*. Before parturition the infant's gut is sterile. The first encounter with micro-organisms occurs in the birth passages of the mother when swallowing of secretions also leads to the swallowing of maternal vaginal flora. Next, when the baby's head appears on the perineum some of the maternal faecal flora, chiefly *E. coli*, are ingested and will then colonise the gut. There is experimental evidence to show that the *E. coli* antibody in breast milk is specific against the *E. coli* in maternal intestinal flora. For example, when pregnant women were fed *E. coli* of an unusual nature it was found that within a week the breast milk contained antibodies against the same type of *E. coli*. There was no serum antibody response seen in the mothers, indicating that plasma cells and other antibody-producing cells in the lymphoid tissue of the mother's intestine are sensitised to the bacterial antigens in the gut lumen and then 'home-in' on the mammary gland where they contribute the specific antibody to the milk.

Breast milk also contains large amounts of the C_3 and C_4 components of complement which can be activated by the antibody contained in the IgA of the milk. The activated complement can act on the cell wall of many gram-negative bacteria exposing the contents of the bacterial cell to immunologic attack. An important factor in such an attack is lysozyme, which occurs in breast milk in large amounts, averaging up to 29–39 mg per 100 ml. Thus the antibodies carried in IgA, acting together with complement and lysozyme, can cause lysis of the bacterial cell in the gut lumen.

An iron-binding protein in breast milk, lactoferrin, has been shown to play a key role in the action of IgA on *E. coli*, by inhibiting the proliferation of this organism in the gut of the newborn. Breast milk contains large amounts of lactoferrin – in the region of 2 mg–6 mg/ml. It has a high affinity for ferric iron which *E. coli* require for growth and multiplication. By mopping up the available iron *E. coli* are deprived of it and their growth is slowed. In laboratory experiments it can be demonstrated that in the presence of lactoferrin only traces of antibody are required to cause bacteriostasis. When iron is added, the lactoferrin gets saturated and its action against *E. coli* is lost. Cow's milk has very little lactoferrin – about 0.2 mg/ml. In addition, many commercial preparations have iron added to them, which would encourage the colonisation of the gut with *E. coli*.

The overall effects of the above-mentioned immune factors is to prevent gut colonisation with *E. coli*. In the breast-fed infant the lactobacilli and lactic acid streptococci predominate in the stools as compared to mixed flora and *E. coli* in the infant fed on cow's milk or artificial milk formulae. The composition of breast milk with its high lactose content, low phosphate and low protein provides the correct substrate for the growth of lactobacilli. In addition, breast milk contains the bifidus factor which promotes the growth of lactobacilli so that in laboratory experiments human milk has been found to be 40 to 100 times as effective as cow's milk in supporting the growth of these organisms.

Human milk also contains a large number of cells varying in number from 2000 to 4000/cu mm. These cells are of two main types — the lymphocyte and the macrophage. The lymphocytes are immunologically active and synthesise IgA as well as BIC complement. They are the same cells that 'home-in' on the mammary gland after being sensitised to bacterial antigens in the mother's gut and secrete a specific antibody against these bacteria. The phagocytes of breast milk are capable of destroying klebsiella organisms *in vitro*, and in animal models which were appropriately stressed by hypoxia they were shown to protect against necrotising enterocolitis.

The various defence factors described above act as an immunologic system which prevents the colonisation of the infant's gut with *E. coli* and instead promotes colonisation by lactobacilli. The *E. coli* harboured in the gut of an artificially fed baby constitute a reservoir of potential pathogens. The exact conditions under which they can cause disease is not understood. Their virulence may be related to capsular antigens, or to their ability to adhere to the cells of the gut mucosa prior to invasion, or to their capacity to produce toxins. The immune factors in breast milk will keep the number of *E. coli* in the gut low until such time as the baby has developed his own immunity. In this way breast milk is unique in its importance, being an agent which protects at the same time as it nurtures, and the mammary gland performs a function not very different from that of the placenta in intrauterine life.

Closely related to protection from infection is the role of human milk in preventing hypersensitivity especially with regard to atopic disease. In families with a strong history of hypersensitivity it is often found that the offspring have transient IgA deficiency in the first few months of life. Secretory IgA in the gut lumen is known to prevent the adsorption of antigen on the mucosal cells of the gut villi. When there is a deficiency of IgA macromolecules of antigen in the gut lumen are able to pass through the cells and enter the blood stream or lymphatics and trigger an immune response. It is postulated that breast milk with its high content of IgA prevents the escape of antigen into the blood stream and thus protects against atopic disease. On the other hand, cow's milk or preparations based on it provide the body with a foreign protein in high concentration. Analyses of samples of ileo-caecal fluid in breast-fed infants show that up to the age of 10 days, 1.3 per cent protein is the maximum concentration at which the protein is completely digested and assimilated. The tolerance for higher concentration rises gradually so that at 3 to 5 months the infant can handle a feed containing protein at 2.5 per cent concentration. Many commercial preparations contain protein at a much higher concentration than this, as shown in the table below.

Milk	Protein calories as % of total calories
Breast milk	7.0
Cow & Gate 1	18.3
Cow & Gate 2	21.9
Cow & Gate Formula	12.2
Cow & Gate Trufood	12.5
Ostermilk 1	16.1
Ostermilk 2	21.6
Ostermilk complete formula	10.5
Golden Ostermilk	21.6
S.M.A.	9.7

The foregoing description of the mechanisms of secretion of breast milk is to emphasise the biological fact that the synthesis and secretion of the main constituents of milk by the alveolar cell of the mammary gland are under the influence of the genetic information carried in the cell nucleus and are specific to the species, and may even be specific to each mother—child pair. For the offspring the milk of its mother is the biological true food. No amount of 'adjusting' can turn the milk of one mammal into a biologically suitable food for the offspring of the other. The history of the baby food industry is full of examples where modifications led to products which gave rise to deficiencies in the infant. Some of these, like pyridoxine deficiency, haemolytic anaemia and electrolyte load, have already been mentioned. There is of course physiological flexibility in every living being, and within limits there is a margin of safety, so that excess or deficiency or alteration in the chemical nature of a nutrient may be tolerated by the infant. And this explains why it has been possible to feed babies on cow's milk and on formulae based on it. But such artificial feeding carries risks. Infants who are fed artificially are biologically different from those who are breast-fed. Their blood carries a different pattern of amino acids, some of which may be at levels high enough to cause anxiety. The composition of their body fat is different. They are fed a variety of carbohydrates to which no other mammalian offspring is exposed in neonatal life. They have higher plasma osmolality, urea and electrolyte levels. Their guts are colonised by a potentially invasive type of microflora, at the same time as they are exposed to large amounts of foreign proteins resulting in an immunologic response. In addition, they are deprived of the various immune factors present in human breast milk. All these factors need to be taken into consideration every time a decision is made not to breast-feed an infant, for inherent in such a decision are known and unknown risks for the infant. Certainly, in those instances where the physiologic reserves of the infant are low, or have been compromised as in pre-term babies, those who have suffered hypoxia, in cases of major surgery and in stresses of all forms, feeding with the mother's milk should be considered obligatory.

Further Reading

1. B. Mepham, *The Secretion of Milk*. Studies in Biology No. 68 (London: Arnold, 1976).
2. A. T. Cowie and J. S. Tindal, *The Physiology of Lactation* (London: Arnold, 1972).
3. J. L. Linzell and M. Peaker, 'Mechanism of Milk Secretion', *Physiological Review* 51, 564 (1971).

Chapter 5

Artificial Feeding of Infants—
a Historical Review

All traditional societies recognise the importance of breast milk for the survival of the infant. A variety of customs and practices can be found in many village communities for the stimulation and promotion of milk secretion in the parturient woman. These include the eating of specially prepared foods for the mother, potions made from herbs and roots which are believed to possess lactagogue properties, massage and hot fomentation of the breasts, in addition to regular suckling by the infant. The Papyrus Ebers, which was dated about 1550 B.C., contains a small paediatric section which includes: 'To get a supply of milk in a woman's breast for suckling a child: Warm the bones of a swordfish in oil and rub her back with it. Or let the woman sit cross-legged and eat fragrant bread of soured dura, while rubbing the parts with the poppy plant.'

Anthropological literature is full of descriptions of how peasant societies cope with the infant for whom mother's milk is not available because of illness or death. The commonest way is for such an infant to be fed by a close relative within the extended family system or within the clan. Usually it is a woman who is breast feeding an infant of her own, but there are now several recorded instances of the maternal grandmother putting the infant to the breast and being able to produce milk. Margaret Mead has cited instances in the villages of Java where the infant was breast-fed by the deceased woman's sister, even though in several cases such a sister had not borne a child before and was a virgin.

In the fifteenth- and sixteenth-century writings in Western Europe there is very little mention of artificial feeding, and breast feeding has been emphasised. For example in *The Nursing of Children*, written by Jacques Gillemeau, a leading French obstetrician, and translated into English in 1612, it is stated: 'There is no difference between a woman who refuses to nurse her own childe, and one that kills her childe as soon as she has conceived.' Half a century later, in 1662, Elizabeth Clinton, the Dowager Countess of Lincoln, wrote a short book called *Countesse of Lincolne's Nurserie*, where she emphasised 'the duty of nursing, due by mothers to their own children'. The countess had eighteen children, none of whom she breast-fed. All but one died in infancy. When the wife of the only surviving son breast-fed her child and he thrived, the mother-in-law was smitten with remorse and said in her book that 'dry breasts were a confession of past wickedness'.

In Tudor England the duration of breast feeding was about two years and by the beginning of the twentieth century it was about nine months. In the context of the social and medical scene of those times breast feeding was probably the most important factor in infant survival. In the year 1863 a report from the Children's Hospital in Manchester showed that whereas 62.6 per cent of the breast-fed infants could be described as well-developed, in the 'hand-reared' group the proportion was only 10 per cent. The *Lancet,* in 1878, pointed out that 69 per cent of deaths in hand-reared legitimate infants and 68 per cent of deaths in hand-reared illegitimate infants were due to diarrhoea, whereas for suckled infants the proportions were 45 per cent and 43 per cent respectively. These figures are very similar to those of the developing countries today.

Breast feeding was not universal all over Western Europe. Sharp regional variations were known to exist in Bavaria in 1905. There were provinces where the majority of the children were never breast-fed, and there were other provinces where almost all were breast-fed. Similarly, an analysis in 1900 of a large number of reports from all regions of Austria showed that it was common practice not to breast-feed infants in those areas of Austria which border on eastern and southern Bavaria. This custom of not breast feeding the infant was a long-established tradition dating back to the fifteenth and sixteenth centuries. There are several reports which show that in the fifteenth century it was common in southern Bavaria to feed the infants meal pap instead of breast milk, and the custom was so firmly established that social disapproval and pressures were brought to bear on the few mothers who may decide to nurse their infants. The statistics of Baden between 1880 and 1900 show that the proportion of children never breast-fed remained constant at 20 per cent. In Berlin there was a considerable change in breast-feeding practice between 1885 and 1905, and the percentage of children under the age of one year who were breast-fed declined from 74.3 per cent to 56.2 per cent.

THE WET NURSE

In the fifteenth- and sixteenth-century writings there is little mention of artificial feeding of infants, so that the custom of offering meal pap to babies in Bavaria is most likely one of the few isolated examples. Animal milk, as a substitute for breast milk, was used in rare cases, and the only alternative, when mother's milk was not available, was the milk of another woman, viz. the wet nurse.

The wet nurse was firmly established in the Western tradition. It is known that in Homeric Greece (950 B.C.) wet nurses were in frequent demand, particularly by women of higher social class. They were given due importance in the household and held positions of authority and responsibility over the servants and slaves, and often continued to look after their charges until adolescence. In the Ptolemic period the Greek influence resulted in an increased use of slaves as wet nurses who usually breast-fed their charges for six months or longer and then used cow's milk. In Roman times wet nurses were common and many of the medical writers of the time comment on the attributes and qualities to be looked for in the wet nurse, the foods she should eat, and the kind of life she should lead in order to secrete adequate quantities of wholesome milk.

The eighteenth century was the peak period for wet nurses in Europe. Ladies of quality did not breast-feed because it was unfashionable, and feared that it may injure their health or ruin their figures, but above all, because it interfered with social rounds or official duties. At the time of the birth of the Prince of Wales (later George IV) in England in 1762, the official announcement included, 'Wet-nurse, Mrs. Scott, Dry-nurse, Mrs. Chapman, Rockers — James Simpson and Catherine Johnson. . . .' In France wet nurses were well-organised from the twelfth century onwards and by 1715 four employment agencies existed in Paris for the registration of nurses, who were required to give their name, age and details of the physical condition of their baby. In order to safeguard the interest of the infants of the wet nurses a law was passed in 1762 which forbade a nurse from taking charge of an infant unless her own was older than 9 months. The legislation also provided for regular medical inspection of the nurses.

The health profession was closely involved in the use of wet nurses in several ways. The medical writings of the time helped to evolve the principles on which the selection of such nurses was based. Individual physicians maintained a register of wet nurses, the 'nurse-book', and made recommendations on establishing the standard rates of pay for the nurses. They also helped the families under their care to make the appropriate choice. Much of the advice was, of course, based on empirical considerations (e.g. mental and personality traits of the nurse passing on to the infant through suckling), and on information that had been passed on from one textbook to another since the Greco-Roman times. There were also others who made detailed observations on the milk output and the growth of the infants. Chief among this latter group of physicians was Pierre Budin of Paris whose book *The Nursling* was a standard reference text at the time and was translated into

English in 1907. At the 'Maternité' in Paris he was the first to demonstrate that a reliable assessment of the output of milk can be made by weighing the infant accurately before and after a feed. He made observations on 14 wet nurses who were assigned 40 infants to feed between them in addition to their own. Each was providing an average of 34 feeds per day and the daily output of milk varied from 1657 g to 2230 g. His observations and teaching helped to establish the study of human lactation on a scientific basis.

The practice of wet nursing also gave rise to several abuses. It offered a lucrative employment to young women from the poorer classes, who managed to get themselves pregnant and then 'overlaid' or 'lost' the infant in order to find employment in a well-to-do household as a wet nurse. This contributed not only to permissiveness but also to high infant mortality. It was not uncommon to find abandoned children on the streets of many of the large cities, and their plight aroused public conscience. Moreover, it was now widely known that venereal infection, especially syphilis, could be transmitted to the infant by his wet nurse. Several literary figures of the time, Addison and Swift among them, and leaders of the Church, campaigned against the use of the wet nurse and in support of breast feeding by the mother. In a book published in 1863 with the title *Infant Feeding and its Influence on Life* the author speaks out against the moral disadvantage of employing wet nurses as 'familiarizing our house-hold with the spectacle of vice rewarded' and warned about 'the master, mistress and other servants becoming tainted by these fallen women'. In spite of such outcries and campaigns against some of the evils of wet nursing, no less than 270 dead infants were found on the streets of London in the year 1870. In the same year the Infant Life Protection Society was founded.

It is curious that a practice which provided for the care and nourishment of the infants of the well-to-do led to such neglect and misery in infants of the poorer classes. Many such children were taken over by the parish, but the mortality among them was very high. Jonas Hanway in his *Journal of Eight Days' Journey* published in 1757 had estimated that only 1 in 70 such children entrusted to the parish survived to grow to adulthood, 'thence to be sent out into the streets to beg, steal or become prostitutes'. Closely related to the practice of wet-nursing was that of 'baby-farming', where fashionable families sent their babies to women in the country who soon neglected their charges. In 1872 a select committee's report to the House of Commons inspired an Act of Parliament which tightened up the regulations with respect to infants under the age of one year kept for gain. This Act brought to an end the practice of baby-farming, which was estimated to result in a mortality of 60 per cent.

The tide of social opinion was turning against the wet nurses not only on moral and religious grounds, but also because some of their practices were shown to be dangerous. Many medical writings of the nineteenth century warn parents against the ill effects of these practices. It used to be common for wet nurses to give 'malt liquor' to the babies in order to make them fat. Some used to sedate their charges with opium derivatives to keep them quiet, and some would cause addiction in the infant by regular application of laudanum to their nipples.

Towards the end of the nineteenth century wet nurses were rarely employed in England, although in France and Russia they were part of the regular staff of the foundling hospitals. In the early years of the twentieth century the use of wet nurses diminished to vanishing-point even on the continent of Europe, but, because of the well-recognised importance of breast milk, milk banks for expressed breast milk were established in several large cities. The first such milk bank was opened in Boston in 1910, and the first in London was at Queen Charlotte's Hospital.

USE OF ANIMAL MILK FOR INFANT FEEDING

The use of cow's milk for feeding the older child has been an established practice since ancient times. The establishment of foundling hospitals in several cities of Europe created a need for a suitable method for feeding a large population of infants. The milks of several animal species were studied, both as regards their chemical constituents and also with the microscope. In the nineteenth century it was already known that ass's milk was the closest to human milk as regards the chemical constituents, and in some hospitals in France stables were maintained for asses and goats to supply milk for the infant. Pierre Budin, at the Maternité in Paris, was beginning to use cow's milk, which was more easily available than ass's or goat's milks. He preferred human milk whenever possible, but in its absence would use undiluted, sterilised cow's milk. The milk was given out daily, pre-sterilised and sealed in bottles each containing the approximate amount required for one feed. He was thus able to demonstrate the value of proper sterilisation. In those times it was widely believed that the heating of milk resulted in the loss of vital elements so that all milk was offered fresh and sometimes even suckled by the infant directly from the animal!

A problem with the use of fresh cow's milk in infant feeding was adulteration and an appalling lack of cleanliness. In 1895 an analysis of 30 samples of milk from working-class areas in London revealed that 24 were 'sophisticated', either by the removal of cream to a level below 3 per cent, or by dilution, or by the addition of boric acid. In the following year 101 samples of milk on sale in London were analysed, and in 68 the fat had been skimmed off to the extent of 20 to 30 per cent. In one sample 65 per cent of the fat had been removed. Water had been added to 89 samples, up to the extent of 30 per cent. A similar situation existed in France. In 1897 the milk in 20 districts of Paris was analysed, and it was found that in only 6 cases did the milk have a fat content of 30 g/l., the normal being 40 g/l. In 14 districts the fat content of milk was less than 30 g and in some it was as low as 15 g/l.

Another problem with cow's milk was its digestibility. Early studies and observations had shown that it forms large and tough curds as compared to human milk. A considerable amount of attention was paid to improving the digestibility of the protein of milk. The easiest approach was to reduce the protein content by dilution with water, or barley water, with sugar added. Many paediatricians of the time believed that minute variation in a single food element could make a great deal of difference to the digestibility and food value of the milk, so that milk was being prescribed with the same precision as a drug. A book on infant feeding published in 1904 carried 2½ pages of algebraic formulae for calculating the exact milk requirement of an infant.

Acidification was another method used to improve the digestibility of milk. Lactic, citric or tartaric acids were used for the purpose. In some cases milk was diluted with acidified whey. Tartared whey, citric acid whey and white wine whey were recommended by Still and quoted by Cautley in his *Diseases of Children* in 1910. Cautley also recommended peptonised or predigested milk. Various peptonising powders were being sold, the most popular being 'Allenbury's peptonising powder' and 'Fairchild's peptogenic milk powder', both of which consisted of pancreatin, bicarbonate of soda and milk sugar. Cow's milk treated with such preparations was sold as 'humanised milk'. Yeast fermentation of milk ('Kumys' and 'Matzoon') was also employed for the same reason, though these preparations were more common in the United States. Holt's *Diseases of Infancy and Childhood* published in 1907 gives the formulae for the home preparation of these products. The fermentation resulted in the casein of milk to be coagulated at first, and later to break up into minute particles. The sugar in milk was converted to lactic acid, which gave the product a sour taste and some was fermented into alcohol. Hence these products were mainly used for older children rather than infants.

Condensed milk was introduced in the artificial feeding of infants towards the latter part of the nineteenth century. The process was patented in 1835. Fresh cow's milk was heated to 212°F (100°C) to destroy the bacteria, and then evaporated in a partial vacuum to less than a quarter of the volume into a viscous honey-like substance, which was found to keep longer than ordinary milk. Sugar was added as a preservative in the proportion of 6 ounces to a pint. At first it was sold in wax-capped bottles until 1866 when Nestlé marketed the first condensed milk in tin boxes. It was soon observed that prolonged feeding of infants on condensed milk gave rise to rickets and scurvy, and several paediatric texts written at about that time give a warning of these complications. One of the classical cases of scurvy described by Barlow in 1883 was a boy aged 15 months who had been fed on 'Swiss milk', Robinson's groats, baked flour, condensed milk, Robb's biscuits, Liebig's extract and saccharated lime water in turn since being weaned at the age of six weeks. The popularity of condensed milk and starchy foods together with overcrowded living conditions and the employment of women and children gave rise to the high incidence of rickets in the late nineteenth century.

—Towards the end of the nineteenth century the main commercial use of cow's milk was for the production of cream and butter. Milk separators were being used in Britain by 1885, and cream appeared on the market in large quantities in 1895. The separated milk was usually sold back to the farmers for feeding pigs and calves, and some was sold as 'pudding milk' for use in cooking. The surplus cream was made into butter and sold as such. The easy availability of separated milk and cream in large quantities led to the establishment of milk laboratories which undertook the preparation of feeds for infants. The first such laboratory was set up in Boston in 1892, followed by another in New York in 1893 and after that several cities in the United States and Europe followed suit. These laboratories prepared infant formulae of different compositions on request and supplied them to individuals, foundling homes and hospitals. The main constituents used by the milk laboratories for preparing the feeds were: (i) Cream containing 32 per cent fat. (ii) Skimmed milk from which fat had been removed. (iii) Standard solution of milk sugar of 20 per cent strength. At times whey was added to modify the protein of milk. The pH of the mixture was adjusted by the addition of lime water. Most milk laboratories were also able to add, on request, gruels of wheat, oats or barley 'of any desired strength', and delivered the mixture sterilised and ready to feed.

THE USE OF POWDERED COW'S MILK IN INFANT FEEDING

The roller process for drying milk was first introduced on a commercial scale by the Swedish butter factories. In this process liquid milk is applied as a thin film to the surface of internally heated drums. The heat drives off the water of the milk and the solids are scraped off the surface of the drum as flakes which are then milled into powder. The first machine was introduced in England in 1902 and soon the separated milk, after the removal of cream, was being sold in the powdered form for use in baking and for making puddings. Shortly afterwards the spray-drying process was used in France. Here liquid milk is sprayed into chambers of hot air and the dried solids of milk fall as a fine powder to the base of the chamber. The roller-dried milk is subjected to a greater degree of heat than spray-dried milk, a factor which affects the protein and the digestibility of the powder. Before subjecting the milk to the drying process the fat content was adjusted to provide full-cream, half-cream or non-fat milk powder. It was not long before the market was flooded with a large number of formulae based on variations in the fat, protein and carbohydrate content.

In 1904 reports were published by the Carnegie Laboratory in New York showing the beneficial results of feeding the poor tenement children of that city on dried milk. In the same year the Medical Officer of Health in Leicester, England, used full-cream and later half-cream powdered milk for feeding children of the poorer classes in that city. Advertisements for dried full-cream, half-cream and separated milk were carried in *The Medical Officer* of 3 October 1908, which stated, 'besides the fact of our supplying a number of infant milk depots, crèches and institutions we can produce thousands of letters from doctors and parents testifying to the splendid results from feeding babies on our Dried English Milk . . .'. In 1908 a large quantity of dried milk powder from New Zealand was marketed in Britain and sold under the brand name of 'Glaxo'. Its introduction coincided with the development of the infant welfare clinics and 'Glaxo' was made available in the clinics at about half the price in the shops. The sales of 'Glaxo' grew as the number of clinics increased.

Efforts were continuing to produce a form of powdered milk which would resemble human milk in its chemical composition. Some of these were made possible by an improved understanding of human nutrition and by technological advances. For example, when the vitamins A, B and C were identified and their synthesis in the laboratory was achieved in the 1920s, most of the leading manufacturers of milk powders began to add these vitamins to their products by 1931. At the same time several products of doubtful value also appeared on the market. In 1919 a formula was promoted under the proprietary name of Scientific Milk Adaptation (S.M.A. for short) in which the fat of cow's milk was replaced by a mixture of cod liver oil and tallow, chosen so that the iodine value of the fat was the same as that of human milk fat. This preparation was selling until 1935, when it was shown that the fat in it was poorly absorbed by the infant's gut. In addition, calcium and phosphorus formed soaps with the unabsorbed fat and were also lost as such. Scientific Milk Adaptation was the forerunner of many more recent products presently being advertised as having a fat composition similar to that of human milk. In all the recent formulae the fat of cow's milk is replaced by a mixture of vegetable oils like coconut, cottonseed and soya oil. Some also contain oleo oils which are destereanated beef fat.

Attempts are also continuing to adjust the protein content of the powdered milks. All of them suffer the same disadvantages as cow's milk, on which they are based. The proteins contained in the whey of cow's milk were known to be better digested by the infant as compared to the protein of casein. As we have seen, whey was used in various forms to 'humanise' cow's milk at the beginning of the century. With the growth of the cheese industry, in which whey is a by-product, the producers of cheese were left with large quantities of whey on their hands and its disposal became a burden. Sites for the dumping of whey were set up, but still the removal of whey to these sites meant considerable labour and transport costs. Some commercial demand for whey was provided by its use in the feeding of livestock and pigs, and many manufacturers of cheese found it commercially attractive to operate pig farms as suitable outlets for the surplus whey. A breakthrough came with the use of whey in the manufacture of baby foods. The final product had a low-protein content and the amino-acid composition resembled that of human milk more closely than in the case of whole milk powder (Figs 5.1, 5.2, 5.3). A new generation of powdered 'milks' has now emerged which are based on whey from which excess electrolytes are removed by dialysis. To this low-electrolyte whey are added a mixture of vegetable fats, and sugars of

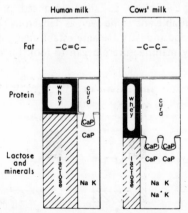

—Composition of human and cows' milk. Cows' milk contains more protein (mainly curd protein), more minerals (some of which form micellar complexes with protein), less lactose, and about the same quantity of fat (but of different quality) when compared with breast milk.

FIG. 5.1 Humanising cow's milk

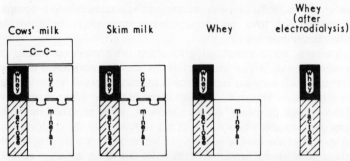

Cows' milk   Skim milk   Whey   Whey (after electrodialysis)

Products of dairy industry which are used in manufacture of infant formulae: whole cows' milk; skim milk (a byproduct of butter manufacture); whey, consisting of whey protein, lactose, minerals, and water (a byproduct of cheese manufacture) and whey demineralised by electrodialysis.

FIG. 5.2   Humanising cow's milk

various sorts to produce a modern version of 'humanised' milk. Thus the humanisation of cow's milk has an interesting history, beginning with dilution by the addition of water or whey, followed in later years by peptone digestion of casein, finally ending in more recent times with the introduction of products which are in effect a mixture of whey proteins, sugars and vegetable oils with added minerals and vitamins. Each generation of 'humanised' milk was promoted in its time as the most advanced form of infant feeding. In fact each product was as advanced as the technology and the knowledge of nutrition at the time. As knowledge grew, many so-called advanced products had to be discarded as unsuitable and some even as dangerous (Fig. 5.4).

As the baby-food industry became established, competition became intense and many manufacturers began to look for export markets. As

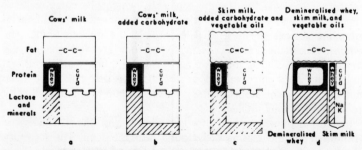

Modifications of whole cows' milk (a) in manufacture of infant formulae; (b) added carbohydrate; (c) substituted fat; and (d) demineralised whey.

FIG. 5.3   Humanising cow's milk

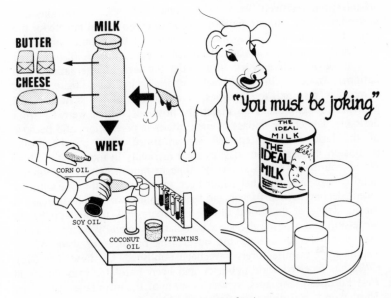

FIG. 5.4   Ideal baby food

early as 1928 Special Export Milk Food was introduced by a British manufacturer as 'suitable for use in the tropics', followed by Sprulac in 1931. Both these products were aimed at Britons living abroad as officials and civil servants in the colonial governments and as members of the Diplomatic Corps. Because of their position as the élite and trend-setters in the colonial society they were the natural targets for the promoters of baby foods. A bewildering number of products appeared with allegedly special properties described by their brand names like Frailac (for premature babies), Allergilac, Sprulac, Humanised Milk Food, etc. The competition became less intense during the Second World War, but began to heat up again in the 1950s when the industrialised world recovered from the after-effects of the war. At this time many of the larger manufacturers began to recruit personnel for the promotion of their products and developed sales training schools. As the number of such trained personnel with special skills grew, the manufacturers were able to expand their sales at home and, later, to launch promotion campaigns on a global scale. Mounting profits enabled many companies to grow into strong multinational corporations.

Birth rates in Western Europe and North America were beginning to decline in the fifties, after a short-lived 'baby boom' in the immediate post-war period. The Third World with its growing populations, rapid urbanisation, relatively weak professional and social institutions and understaffed government departments became the logical targets for the promoters of infant foods. Moreover, many of the populations of the developing world had already been sensitised to the use of powdered milk through its free distribution under the aegis of international and national agencies. In their zeal for improving sales figures some companies resorted to activities, like the use of 'milk nurses' and provision of 'gift packs' in maternity hospitals, which were far from desirable. Under the impact of such intensive promotion, and because of the lack of a united and well-informed stand by the health profession, breast feeding has declined markedly in most of the Third World countries (Fig. 5.5). At no time in human history has such a rapid change in human behaviour been recorded as is the case with the recent decline in breast feeding in the developing world. The increase in the incidence of diarrhoeal disease and marasmus alarmed the health profession and aroused the social conscience in many Western societies. Several reports describing the advertising practices of some of the leading milk manufacturers have been published. Of these, *The Baby Killer* has received wide publicity and been translated into almost all West European languages, as well as some of the main languages of the Third World. A German translation which carried a provocative title led to a libel suit in a Swiss court, in which one major manufacturer of baby foods came under strong criticism.

The arousing of social conscience in Western societies, very much

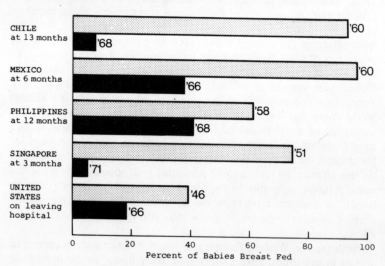

FIG. 5.5   Decline in breast feeding in some developing countries

like that in the eighteenth century, has helped to generate a great deal of interest in the scientific and social aspects of breast feeding. In the meantime many of the more humane manufacturers of baby milks have declared a moratorium against the promotion of their own products by unfair means. On their part the governments of several developing countries have introduced legislation against the advertising of milk powders. Such legislation, however belated, will go a long way towards laying the foundation of the social legislation so necessary for the proper evolution of infant welfare movements.

Further Reading

1. I. Wickes, 'History of Infant Feeding', *Arch. Dis. Childh.* **28**, 151, 232, 332, 416, 495 (1953).
2. M. Muller, *The Baby Killer*, 2nd edn (London: War on Want, 1975).
3. Editorial article 'The Infant Food Industry', *Lancet* **2**, 503 (1976).

Chapter 6

Breast Feeding and the Third World

Two-thirds of the world's population lives in the Third World. In the average developing country up to 80 per cent or more of the population is rural, living in either scattered homesteads or in small villages and hamlets. Of the 20 per cent or so living in larger towns and cities more than a fifth live in crowded tenements and shanty towns. The existing rural health services are stretched to their limit so that less than 20 per cent of the rural population receives any basic health care on a regular basis. Curative services in the form of hospitals in urban areas absorb more than three-quarters of the total health budget. In spite of the concentration of the health professionals in the cities the weaker sections of the urban population in slums and shanty towns do not enjoy any better health facilities than their counterparts in rural areas. At present several innovative approaches in health care are being developed by a number of countries in order to extend basic health care to all sections of the population and to rectify the present inequality in health care. The success of these efforts remains to be seen.

Only a quarter to a third of the population in an average developing country is literate. Primary school education and adult literacy campaigns are given high priorities in all Third World countries and take up almost 40 per cent of the total government expenditure. In spite of these efforts progress is slow and the existing rate of illiteracy is a major obstacle to the rapid spread of information, so that there is widespread ignorance, including that of simple hygiene. Because of illiteracy and ignorance traditional beliefs and customs prevail in all developing societies.

Poverty is another major factor, and the resources available to the average family for nutrition, housing and improvement of environment are acutely limited. It is estimated that up to 40 per cent of the population of the average developing country exists below the bread line. Environmental sanitation is virtually non-existent so that there is high endemicity of water-borne diseases in all rural communities. The lack of hygiene, poor nutrition, lack of clean water, inadequate health facilities, widespread ignorance and a traditional attitude act together to perpetuate a vicious spiral of disease and death.

The feeding and rearing of infants in the Third World should be viewed against this background of the environmental, social and disease situation.

THE RURAL SOCIETY

Breast feeding is the normal way of feeding infants in all peasant societies. In a world-wide study of 45 different cultural and ethnic groups it was found that on average the infant is breast fed for 1½ to 2 years, though 4 years was not very uncommon and in some communities it may continue for as long as 6 years. In such a cultural setting the average child grows up to consider breast feeding as the natural way of rearing infants. The extended family system, and the close communal life of the village, present continuing opportunities for the young to observe the dynamics of breast feeding, and the average adolescent grows up with a positive attitude towards lactation.

Marriages tend to occur early in most peasant communities and normally take place about the time of menarche. In several studies the average age at marriage in the case of the female has been found to be between 10 and 14 years. Consequently, the age of the mother at the time of first delivery is also young, and has been reported as between 15 and 18 years in such studies (Table 6.1). The young mother is likely to be full of anxieties and fears, and derives a great deal of comfort and confidence from the womenfolk of the extended family and the kin group.

TABLE 6.1   Age at marriage and first delivery in Hyderabad, India

Area	No.	Age at marriage					
		Age (years)					
		−7	7−10	10−12	12−14	14−16	16+
Rural 1	100	—	12	18	32	30	8
Rural 2	300	9	69	141	67	12	2
Urban	100	—	4	2	16	46	18

Area	No.	Age at first delivery			
		Age (years)			
		−16	16−18	18−20	20+
Rural	100	28	44	20	8
Urban	100	10	48	22	20

(Adapted from G. J. Ebrahim, 'Cross-cultural Aspects of Breast Feeding', in *Breast Feeding and the Mother*, Ciba Foundation Symposium No. 45 (1976))

The birth of the baby is supervised by the traditional birth attendant, helped by the elder women of the immediate family. Together they ensure that the traditional practices are observed and the various rituals are carried out in every minute detail. The baby and the mother are isolated from all outside contacts for the period of the puerperium, which can vary from 21 to 40 days in different cultures. In many cases the mother is also immobilised during this period and is not expected to take on any household duties. Such a period of enforced isolation and immobilisation as part of the ritual throws the mother and her baby together and helps to sensitise them to each other. During this period of isolation the birth attendant visits the mother several times daily to massage her body with oil, to bathe the baby and to help with some of the household chores. She also gives advice on simple problems, especially those relating to the feeding of the baby. She is thus both a source of advice and comfort to the mother and throughout this very sensitive period helps to cushion her against anxiety. This role of the birth attendant in providing advice and information when needed, and allaying maternal anxiety within the cultural environment in which the mother and her baby are isolated from outside influences, is crucial in the establishment of lactation. In a study of several cultures this function of 'mothering the mother' stands out as the most important factor in the proper establishment of breast feeding. Such a supportive role of the birth attendant as apart from acting as a midwife is now being described by the term 'doula'. Many observers have confirmed the important contribution of the 'doula' in getting breast feeding established during the sensitive period of the puerperium (Fig. 6.1).

The health plans of all Third World countries recognise the importance of maternity services, especially in rural areas. As these services have grown, more and more women have come forth to make use of the facilities offered by the health centres. They receive better midwifery care during labour, but the trained nurses and midwives have so far been incapable of performing the functions of the 'doula'. Instead the experience so far indicates that mothers in the average maternity unit are easy targets for advertising with wall posters and photographs, visits by the 'milk nurses' and issues of gift packs. Some of the practices of the maternity unit, copied from the obstetric department of the teaching hospital, like separation of the baby from the mother or offering bottle feeds at night or as prelacteal feeds, may act against the smooth establishment of breast feeding. It is obvious that unless these weaknesses of 'modernised' obstetric care can be rectified and the training of the health personnel be made more relevant to rural needs, growth of obstetric services may well turn out to have an adverse effect on breast feeding. As the 'doula' gets displaced by trained

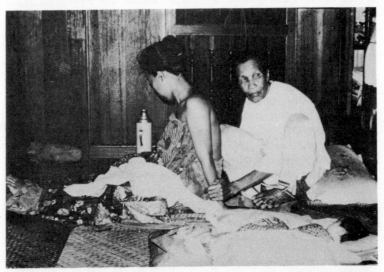

FIG. 6.1   The traditional birth attendant who visits daily to massage the mother with oil, bathe the baby and provide emotional support during the period of puerperal isolation

midwives and nurses at the health centre, or by auxiliaries and trained birth attendants in smaller hamlets, it will be important to ensure that some of the weaknesses of present-day midwifery do not spread and cause a decline in breast feeding.

THE URBAN SOCIETY

The cities of the developing world house the small but important group of the urban élite, consisting of industrialists, businessmen, professionals, administrators and political leaders. Many of them enjoy living standards as high as those of similar groups in the affluent societies of the West. But there is one important difference. The urban élite of the Third World constitute a key group in the social, political and financial affairs of the nation. They are the trend-setters of the developing world. The physicians and other health professionals who look after this 'modern sector' are keen to suggest and promote practices which will be considered trendy and modern. The tendency for bottle feeding in the Third World springs largely from this so-called modern sector.

The vast majority of the urban population, however, consists of the poorest segments of the country's population who are new migrants to the city and inhabit the inner city areas, the slums and the shanty towns. In many cases the urban poor are a result of the overflow of the rural poverty into the cities. With the increase in population in rural areas the worse-off families form a continuing stream of migrants into the cities. As such they constitute one of the most deprived social groups in a country. They leave behind their social and cultural values and come to adopt a rootless existence. Since the urban system is geared to the life-styles of the urban élite, these families come under the influence of the new trends and the temptation to mimic the practices of the élite is very strong (Fig. 6.2). Many work in the homes of the upper social classes as house servants and child-minders, where they come to observe a different way of feeding infants out of cans. In addition, they also come under the influence of the mass media for the first time, and are barraged with seductive displays through neon signs, placards, posters, radio and television commercials, as well as door-to-door sales personnel. Their children grow up in the hurly burly of life in tenements and shanty towns and absorb very little, if any, of the social values and culture of the parents. On achieving adulthood many women are unprepared for their role as mothers, unlike their counterparts in rural areas. There are no effective means of person-to-person education with regard to breast feeding, as happens in the rural society. There are

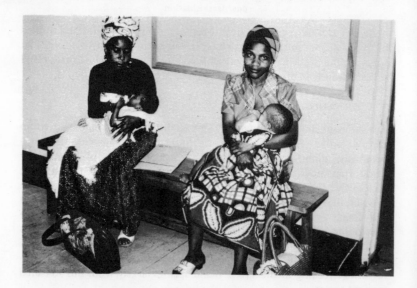

FIG. 6.2   Bottle and breast feeding in a developing society

Note the dress, the expensive handbag and other signs of modernisation in the mother who is bottle feeding.

no national campaigns for the promotion of breast feeding and the paediatric and obstetric services may be too curative in outlook to be effective in the community. In addition, if the mother also happens to be in employment there is no legislation to allow her sufficient length of maternity leave or 'nursing breaks' during the day to feed her infant. The cumulative effect of all these factors has been that more and more mothers are giving up breast feeding.

The post-war years brought a major nutrition intervention programme in many developing countries in the form of free distribution of powdered skimmed milk donated by various international agencies. The programme was conceived with the best of intentions and was based on the experience of the milk depots during the early years of the infant welfare movement in Europe and the United States. Availability of free milk attracted mothers to the maternal and child health clinics and improved the utilisation of services. The programme received professional backing and political support, but it also gave rise to dependence and contributed to the trend of artificial feeding. In some countries, such as Chile, the distribution of powdered milk became an important tool in electioneering and the political leaders made promises of greater coverage of families with free milk during their campaigns. As more families became the beneficiaries of the programme breast feeding declined further. Among the factors that have contributed to the decline of breast feeding in the Third World the free distribution of powdered milk must also take its own share of the blame.

Rural migration as a social phenomenon is now fully established in all Third World countries, and several of them in South America have seen a dramatic change in the distribution of their population. Chile is an extreme example of this phenomenon, where 80 per cent of the population is now urban. Whether this trend can be halted by the present emphasis on rural improvement in the national development plans of many countries remains to be seen. In the meantime unplanned urban growth will continue, giving rise to a staggering number of the urban poor in whom the traditional values are being rapidly eroded and a new slum culture is taking over. Table 6.2 provides data on the growth of some of the major cities of the Third World between 1950 and 1975 and looks at the population figures expected in the next twenty-five years. It is the new arrivals in the city and the urban poor who are at a maximum risk of taking up bottle feeding as a symbol of modernisation.

Urban life demands skills in budgeting the family income. Many of the new arrivals in the city and the urban poor are not accustomed to this way of life and lack the necessary skills for balancing the household budget. When mothers allow themselves to be persuaded to bottle-feed their infants they have usually not thought of the long-term costs of

TABLE 6.2   Urban growth in the Third World

(population in millions)

	1950	Average annual growth (%)	1975	Average annual growth (%)	2000
Africa					
Cairo	2.4	4.3	6.9	3.6	16.9
Lagos	0.3	8.1	2.1	6.2	9.4
Kinshasa	0.2	9.7	2.0	5.6	7.8
Asia					
Bombay	2.9	3.7	7.1	4.2	19.8
Calcutta	4.5	2.4	8.1	3.7	20.4
Jakarta	1.6	5.1	5.6	4.7	17.8
Karachi	1.0	6.2	4.5	5.4	16.6
Manila	1.5	4.4	4.4	4.3	12.8
Seoul	1.0	8.3	7.3	3.8	18.7
Latin America					
Bogotà	0.7	6.5	3.4	4.2	9.5
Buenos Aires	4.5	2.9	9.3	1.5	13.7
Mexico City	2.9	5.4	10.9	4.4	31.5
Rio de Janeiro	2.9	4.4	8.3	3.4	19.3
São Paulo	2.5	5.7	9.9	3.9	26.0

their decision. The average cost of artificially feeding an infant in a developing country can vary from a quarter to a third of the national minimum wage. In fact, because of the high levels of unemployment many wage-earners accept employment at wages which are far lower than the statutory minimal wage, and the cost of artificially feeding an infant in such a case will be a sizeable portion of the family income, as shown in Table 6.3.

TABLE 6.3   Cost of artificial feeding in the Third World

Country	Minimum wage per week (U.S.$)	Cost of feeding a 6-month-old infant per day (U.S.$)	% of wage
United Kingdom	39.20	1.30	3.3
Burma	5.01	0.81	16.2
Peru	5.60	1.30	23.2
Philippines	9.69	2.59	26.7
Indonesia	5.60	1.62	28.9
Tanzania	7.62	2.44	32.0
India	4.62	1.62	35.1
Nigeria	5.18	2.44	47.1
Afghanistan	2.80	1.62	57.9
Pakistan	5.18	3.23	62.4
Egypt	4.09	2.59	63.3

Economic necessity forces many families to make the tin of powdered milk stretch as much as possible by offering dilute feeds to the infant, with the result that there has been a marked increase in the incidence of marasmus in urban areas. In addition, because of the prevailing insanitary conditions in the 'septic fringe' of the cities, bottle feeding has been associated with a rising incidence of diarrhoeal disease. The hospitals do not have adequate facilities to house all the infants coming to them with dehydration, so that makeshift rehydration units have to be set up on a day-care basis. Much of the criticism of artificial feeding in developing countries is because of its contribution to infantile marasmus and diarrhoeal disease (Fig. 6.3). However, in several public debates the manufacturers have clearly stated that the poverty, ignorance and lack of hygiene prevalent in developing countries is no concern of theirs and that they do not consider them as grounds for modifying their sales promotion activities.

Mother's milk is an important resource for a nation, not only from the biological point of view but also from the economic angle. A decline in breast feeding with a resulting importation of powdered milk can be a serious drain on the foreign exchange reserves of a poor country. For example, it is calculated that a decline of only 20 per cent

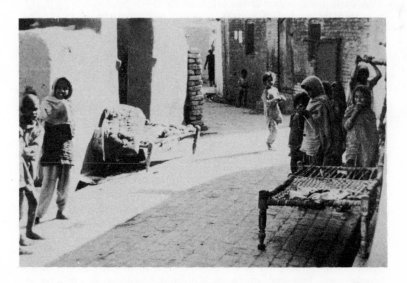

FIG. 6.3   Bottle feeding and its effects in the developing society

Two infants are left with feeding-bottles in a street while their mothers are at work. Fig. 6.3*b* is a close-up of one of the infants.

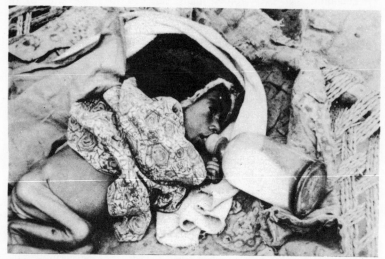

FIG. 6.3b

in breast feeding in Tanzania will require the importation of powdered milk costing £2 million at the prices of 1970. This amount is equivalent to a third of the health budget of the country in 1975, and is equal to the total health budget of Tanzania at the time of independence in 1961. The decline in breast feeding in Chile between 1951 and 1970 is equal to a loss of 78.6 thousand tons of breast milk costing U.S. $18.86 million!

In all future action programmes the role of the health profession will be crucial. Until recently not enough importance has been given to the teaching of the subject in the curricula of the training institutions. Established texts place little emphasis on the subject of breast feeding, and there is virtually no discussion in seminars or tutorials on the social, cultural and economic aspects of infant feeding. To a very considerable extent the medical and nursing professions have allowed themselves to be influenced by the semi-scientific promotional literature put out by the manufacturers of baby foods. Many of the scientific and literary activities of the professional bodies are supported by the manufacturers, which allows the latter to influence the policy decisions of such bodies.

An honest evaluation of the present state of infant nutrition in the country and free dialogue both within the profession and with the manufacturers will allow clear guidelines to be formed. With regard to the role of the health profession in the changing social scene of the Third World countries several studies have demonstrated that the nursing mother has two important needs, viz. detailed information on various aspects of breast feeding and emotional support, especially during the early days of lactation, provided by people in whom she trusts. If these two criteria can be fulfilled in all contacts between the mother and the health personnel she will be more inclined to nurse her baby. A suggested plan of activities that can be performed at different points of contact between the mother and the health service is shown in the table below:

ANTENATAL CLINIC	Information on breast feeding, preferably in group discussion with mothers who are nursing their infants. Information on maternal diet. Preparation of the breasts. Developing positive attitudes towards breast feeding.
LABOUR WARD	Avoidance of unnecessary medication and interventions. Rooming-in with body contact between infant and mother. Avoidance of prelacteal and night-feeds by bottle. Use of lactation advisers, preferably mothers who have breast-fed their infants. Banning of promotion through wall charts, posters, photographs, gift packs and visits from 'milk nurses'.
PREMATURE AND OBSERVATION NURSERY	Use of expressed breast milk. Unrestricted visiting by the mothers.
HOME VISITING	Motivate and support, Provide 'doula' function.
CHILDREN'S WARDS	Accommodation for mothers to stay with their sick infants.
FEMALE WARDS	Accommodation for 'lodger' babies to accompany sick mothers.
UNDER-5 CLINIC	Encourage and support. Avoid issue of milk supplements. Counsel mothers who are bottle-feeding their infants.
GENERAL	Help develop community groups and women's organisations who can disseminate information and create positive attitudes.

There is a need to raise the public's level of awareness with regard to some of the issues surrounding infant feeding. In the West several voluntary organisations like the La Lèche League are providing a valuable service to the people through pamphlets, booklets, public meetings and informal gatherings. Many such national organisations are in close communication with each other and are forming international links. Whenever such organisations have succeeded in obtaining the patronage of the national leaders they have been able to influence the general public more effectively.

Strong voluntary organisations, a committed profession and an informed public can together bring about the necessary pressures to introduce legislation which will safeguard the interests of the infant and the mother. The experience of many of the Western democracies has shown that strong public health and social legislation can help to sow the seeds of the nation's health. Legislation for the prevention of unethical promotion is of course necessary, but equally important is to give to the mother adequate maternity leave and to provide for 'nursing breaks' when she starts work again. Provision of crèches and kindergartens, whether from public funds or voluntary effort, will help to increase the opportunities for the working mother to nurse her child in the middle of a working day. It is only by means of a unified effort at the professional, social and government level that the present rapid decline in breast feeding can be halted in the Third World.

Further Reading

1. C. S. Ford, *A Comparative Study of Human Reproduction*. Publications in Anthropology No. 32 (New Haven, Conn.: Yale University Press, 1945).
2. D. Raphael, *The Tender Gift* (New Jersey, Prentice-Hall, 1973).
3. P. Hakim and G. Solimano, 'Supplemental Feeding as a Nutritional Intervention: the Chilean experience in the distribution of milk', *J. Trop. Paed. Env. Child Health*, Monograph No. 46, **22**, 186 (1976).
4. J. L. Richardson, 'Review of International Legislation Establishing Nursing Breaks', *J. Trop. Paed. Env. Child Health* **21**, 249 (1975).

Index

feeding
  apathy in   32
  difficulties in   31–3
  techniques of   31
feeds
  concentrated   51
  dilute   81

gut, neonatal
  bacterial colonisation of   57
  development of enzymes   20

health attendant, training of   24
Hoffman manoeuvre   26
hormones   8–10

immunoglobulins   55
immunological protection   53

kidney, neonatal   50
kidneys, solute load   49

labour
  effect of sedatives in   19
  local anaesthetics in   19
lactation
  adoptive   24
  and the baby   15
  and the health worker   23
  and maternal nutrition   6
  difficulties in   10, 31–3
  early days of   27
  induced   24
  physiology of   4
  success in   23
  useful hints   31
lactoferrin   57
lactose
  in milk formulae   43
  secretion of   41
learning response   18
let-down reflex   9

mammals   1
mammals, milk of various   2
mammary gland   3
marriage
  age of   75
  in peasant communities   75
milk secretion, mechanisms of   36

nipples
  cracks   32
  protractile   26
nutrition during lactation   5

obesity   50
obstetric practices   28
opinion, public   64, 72
osmolality   50

phosphorus
  in breast milk   52–3
  in cow's milk   52–3
poverty   74
practices
  obstetric, modern   28, 76
  traditional   76
pregnancy, change in body weight
    7, 8
prolactin   9
protein, of human milk   36
protein antigen
  in breast milk   41
  in cow's milk   58–9
psychological aspects   13

reflexes
  let-down   9, 11
  rooting   15
  suckling   16
  swallowing   18
  upper-airway   19
reproduction, central control of
    12, 13
rural society   75

smell, sense of   2, 15
suckling, physiology of   15
synthesis
  of fat   42–3
  of lactose   41
  of protein   37

Third World
  rural population   75
  urban growth   80
  urban population   77
tissue fat, composition of   46
trace metals   51

urine, osmolar load in   49–50

wet nurse, milk output   62
Woolwich method   25